"A must-read for anyone on a he
ability to deeply explore new areas of health before they become trends. I'm so proud of her commitment to becoming an expert in an uncharted territory at a time when we need this kind of support more than ever."

—Gabrielle Bernstein, *New York Times*–bestselling author of *Super Attractor*

"Jenny's courageous and inspiring mission to help her dad through cancer treatments using holistic remedies and plant-based medicine is a topic that's near and dear to my heart. The guidance she shares is a game-changer for patients and caregivers alike."

—Kris Carr, *New York Times*–bestselling author of *Crazy Sexy Diet* and cancer thriver

"Jenny has succeeded in making complex information accessible and practical for self-healing. This book can help pretty much anyone interested in powerful but safe natural approaches to feeling better and living life to its fullest."

—Dr. Dustin Sulak, integrative physician and founder of Healer.com

"*The Rebel's Apothecary* is a delightful, well-informed, user-friendly exploration of the remarkable health benefits of cannabis and medicinal mushrooms. . . . You'll get a big boost from reading this book!"

—Martin A. Lee, director of Project CBD and author of *Smoke Signals*

"When her father was diagnosed with cancer, Jenny Sansouci became a citizen scientist. She diligently poured herself into the research of natural medicine, specifically cannabis and medicinal mushrooms, and the result is *The Rebel's Apothecary*. While not a substitute for appropriate medical care, this book provides two of the important ingredients we need when a loved one is a diagnosed with cancer or a chronic, debilitating, or painful condition: tools to help mitigate their suffering, and possibly improve their immunity, resilience, and health. Help and hope. That's what this book is all about—and who doesn't need that?"

—Aviva Romm, MD, author of *Botanical Medicine for Women's Health* and coeditor of *American Herbal Pharmacopoeia: Cannabis Inflorescence*

"*The Rebel's Apothecary* is very accurate and accessible, written in a clear and folksy style. Many people will benefit from its advice."

"This very important book is the first in the field to combine both cannabis and medicinal mushrooms. *The Rebel's Apothecary* is timely and will be of great interest to a broad readership and also to researchers, mushroom producers, medical doctors, and specialists in alternative medicine. To say this book is unique would be an understatement."

"*The Rebel's Apothecary* is a fantastic resource and the perfect guide for anyone seeking natural and effective strategies to support everyday wellness or relief from insomnia, anxiety, the side effects of chemotherapy, and more. Inspired by her own personal experience, Jenny has transformed her passion into an engaging, step-by-step guide that includes the latest research, protocols, and specific dosing guidelines making the powerful healing possibilities of plant medicine accessible to all."

THE
REBEL's
APOTHECARY

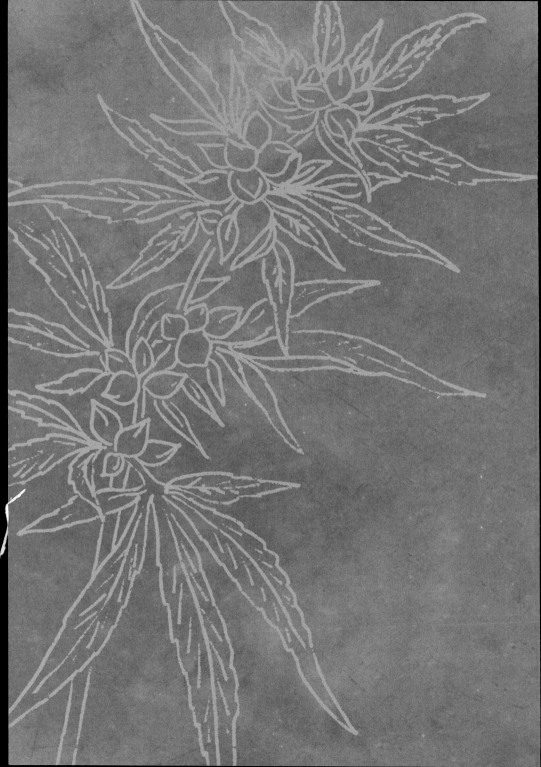

The REBEL's APOTHECARY

A PRACTICAL GUIDE TO THE HEALING MAGIC OF CANNABIS, CBD, AND MUSHROOMS

Jenny Sansouci

Foreword by Frank Lipman, MD

A TARCHERPERIGEE BOOK

TARCHERPERIGEE
an imprint of Penguin Random House LLC
penguinrandomhouse.com

TarcherPerigee with tp colophon is a registered trademark of
Penguin Random House LLC

Most Tarcher/Penguin books are available at special quantity discounts for bulk
purchase for sales promotions, premiums, fund-raising, and educational needs.
Special books or book excerpts also can be created to fit specific needs. For details,
write: SpecialMarkets@penguinrandomhouse.com.

Library of Congress Cataloging-in-Publication Data

Names: Sansouci, Jenny, author. | Lipman, Frank, writer of foreword.
Title: The rebel's apothecary : a practical guide to the healing magic of cannabis,
CBD, and mushrooms / Jenny Sansouci ; foreword by Frank Lipman, MD.
Description: [New York] : TarcherPerigee, an imprint of Penguin Random
House LLC, [2020] | Includes index.
Identifiers: LCCN 2019056755 (print) | LCCN 2019056756 (ebook) | ISBN
9780593086575 (paperback) | ISBN 9780593086582 (ebook)
Subjects: LCSH: Marijuana—Therapeutic use. | Marijuana—Physiological
effect. | Alternative medicine. | Marijuana—Therapeutic use.
Classification: LCC RM666.C266 S26 2020 (print) | LCC RM666.C266 (ebook)
| DDC 615.3/23648—dc23
LC record available at https://lccn.loc.gov/2019056755
LC ebook record available at https://lccn.loc.gov/2019056756

Printed in the United States of America

1 3 5 7 9 10 8 6 4 2

Book design by Lorie Pagnozzi

FOR DAD, MOM, AND LISA.
AND FOR ALL THE CAREGIVERS—
I WROTE THIS FOR YOU.

Contents

THE REBEL'S MANIFESTO

THE REBEL's MANIFESTO

When you hear the words "cannabis" and "mushrooms," the first thought you may have is to equate them with recreational drugs, not medicine. We've been conditioned that way. Thankfully, this perception is evolving, and the therapeutic properties of cannabis and mushrooms (both non-psychedelic *and* psychedelic mushrooms) are becoming widely known. Stories are being shared, research is being conducted, and the medicinal value of these plants and fungi can no longer be ignored.

Conventional medicine, science, and doctors have made huge progress for us as a species, but there are options from the natural world that can supplement our conventional healthcare and enrich our quality of life. In fact, many of the pharmaceutical drugs we use today were originally derived from plants. Conventional medicine can be a wonderful thing—it's just not all there is. This book will introduce you to some of the ways you can use the Earth's gifts for your own healing.

Nature's medicine chest is right outside your door.
It's right under your foot. It's only in the last 100 years or so
that this has fallen away. We are reawakening it now.

—*Cheryl Boiko*

The Rebel's Apothecary isn't about going *against* conventional medicine, pharmaceutical companies, or the legal system. To me, being a "rebel" is about *questioning*. Investigating what you've been taught about health and healing. Doing your own research. Asking "why?" more often. Understanding your options. And most important, *making choices about your body and your health that feel right to you.*

In a world that's feeding us endless processed junk food, pills, and chemicals, it's an act of rebellion to use natural plants and eat natural foods. It's an act of rebellion to take your power back—the power of having a hand in your own well-being.

Being a rebel means having your own opinion. Paying attention to the wisdom from everyone you meet along the way, yet still blazing your own trail. Getting to know your body and what feels good to you. You can take the advice of your doctors, follow conventional wisdom, embrace Western medicine as much as you'd like, *while also adding in gentle but powerful remedies and practices to support every system in your body.*

I don't go first to Western medicine, but thank God
it's there when we need it. Take the best of everything,
at the time that makes sense for you.

—*Jo Anne Richards*

IT'S A REBEL'S JOURNEY TO CREATE
YOUR OWN PATH.

We've been encouraged to listen to only our doctors when it comes to our healthcare—and I believe our doctors are good-intentioned, smart, and genuinely out to help us. But I also believe it's time to get back to our roots—back to the herbs, plants, and fungi that have been available to us and used as potent medicines for healing since the beginning of time.

The information in this book is not to be considered a substitution for your doctor, therapist, or other healthcare professional. I am here, however, to be a messenger—to let you know what your options are in the world of cannabis and medicinal mushrooms, so you can start to ask questions, experiment, and make more informed decisions about your health.

It's time we get back to the ancient practices of using plants as medicine.

I'll help you get started.

It's not rebels that make trouble,

but trouble that makes rebels.

—Ruth Messinger

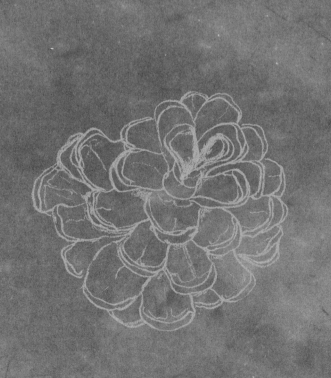

FOREWORD

FRANK LIPMAN, MD

To live a long, healthy, and vital life, I believe in taking an integrative approach. This means using the best that modern medicine has to offer, while supporting well-being through diet, lifestyle, herbs, and supplements. I practice functional medicine, which uses the scientific research, biochemistry, and physiology of Western medicine, along with the ancient healing philosophies of Eastern medicine. The role of functional medicine is to look for the root cause of a problem (rather than only treating the symptoms that arise) in order to improve function, reduce inflammation, and create balance in the body. If you're driving your car and the oil light goes on, you don't just put a Band-Aid over the oil light. You check to see why the oil light went on, and you fix the root of the issue. Ideally, we learn to incorporate daily practices into our lives that prevent that oil light from going on in the first place.

I was trained as a traditional physician in the Western medical system, and while I'm not against Western medicine at all, it has its limitations. Drugs can be helpful, and oftentimes necessary, but many of them are overused and overprescribed. The methods of Western medicine are wonderful for acute care and crisis care. If you break a bone or have appendicitis, a heart attack, or pneumonia, or you need emergency care, Western medicine is appropriate. However, I noticed early on in my days as a conventional M.D. that the problems people suffer from on a day-to-day basis—chronic, low-grade complaints such as fatigue, digestive issues, headaches, stress, insomnia, pain, and anxiety—are issues that Western medicine doesn't really deal with properly.

When I was introduced to acupuncture in 1984, I witnessed how traditional Chinese medicine (which includes the use of plants and herbs) was working well for patients with these everyday health concerns. Traditional Chinese medicine points to an imbalance in the system—you're not simply considered "healthy" or "sick." There's a spectrum. As health practitioners, we're always trying to move people further along the spectrum toward better health. I began to see natural plants, herbs, medicinal mushrooms, acupuncture, and stress-relief techniques as a perfect match for the crisis care that Western medicine provides. I knew the future of medicine would be some kind of combination of the two.

Many cultures throughout history have used plants, herbs, and fungi for health and longevity. Both cannabis and medicinal mushrooms can have tremendous benefits for not only everyday wellness but for staying healthy as we age. Mushrooms are powerful medicines that have been shown to improve brain function and strengthen immunity. I have always used mushrooms in my practice with patients to balance the immune system, because that is the Chinese medicine tradition.

We're just starting to tap into the vast therapeutic potential of cannabis. I work with a lot of stressed-out New Yorkers, and I've seen incredible results with CBD for sleep, relaxation, and anxiety. It really helps people to chill out when they're overstressed. I've also seen patients experience amazing results with CBD for inflammation and skin problems. Cannabis is a wonderful medicine that has so many potential benefits.

Jenny Sansouci is one of my favorite health coaches of all time, and I'm thrilled that you have the opportunity to learn from her in this book. Jenny worked as a health coach in my practice in New York City for four years, and she has worked directly with hundreds of my patients. What I loved about working so closely with Jenny is that she's really good with people—I was always impressed by how much she cared about what each patient was dealing with. She explored every question a patient asked so thoroughly, and if she didn't know about something a patient was struggling with, she'd do everything she could to research it.

The Rebel's Apothecary is an exact reflection of how Jenny worked in my practice. You can trust her to be a reliable source who's done her research and looked at all of the information responsibly. This book is necessary in the world we live in now, where it can be confusing and overwhelming to know where to turn when it comes to our health and wellness.

The right blend of conventional medicine and herbal medicine can help you to feel better every day and live a longer, healthier, more vibrant life. I'm excited to see what will happen with both cannabis and mushrooms in the future, as I believe they are the perfect antidote for the Western ways of living. This book is on the cutting edge of that research.

INTRODUCTION

I f you'd told me a few years ago that I'd be writing a book about cannabis and mushrooms, I wouldn't have believed you. I never imagined I'd become so passionate about these plants (well, plants and
fungi—technically, mushrooms aren't plants). I always equated them
with the "recreational" use I experimented with in college. The terms
"weed" and "shrooms" immediately brought me back to visions of
being surrounded by clouds of pot smoke, giggling and having the
munchies—and the vivid psychedelic experiences I had on mushrooms
while studying abroad.

In 2007, as a twenty-four-year-old party girl who needed to clean
up her life, I quit drinking and swore off all drugs—which, of course,
included cannabis and mushrooms. I never thought I'd have a reason
to revisit them. As I slowly learned to navigate my new drug-free and
alcohol-free existence, I became an explorer of wellness, an avid researcher, and a dedicated experimenter. I started my first blog in 2008
to share what I was learning, and I've been writing online about wellness ever since. I became certified as a health coach through the Institute for Integrative Nutrition in 2010, and worked as a health coach in
Dr. Frank Lipman's functional medicine practice in New York City.
My mind was opened up to new natural remedies daily. Working with
his patients, researching their conditions, and witnessing their improve-

ments showed me the power that dietary changes, lifestyle shifts, herbs, and supplements can have on our well-being.

For more than a decade now, I've been living my passion for wellness and creating a career out of it—but as it turns out, sometimes our greatest sense of purpose can come from the most difficult life experiences.

In 2017, the day before Thanksgiving, the man I look up to most in the world—my dad, my hero—was diagnosed with stage IV pancreatic cancer. My whole family was together in the hospital, and we got the news at the same time. If you've had a loved one diagnosed with cancer, you understand how disorienting that moment feels. Hearing a diagnosis like that is one of the most painful things in the world, and we were immediately overwhelmed by feelings of desperation, hopelessness, and fear.

After the initial shock subsided, I jumped into action mode. When you do an online search for "pancreatic cancer," the majority of what you'll find isn't positive. I resisted the negative information I found with every rebellious beat of my heart—I knew there had to be *something* I could do to help my dad. Suddenly, my passion for wellness was no longer about kale salads and green juice—this was about life or death.

My priority became laser-focused as I dove deeply into what would be the most important and meaningful research of my life. Little did I know, my dad's diagnosis would catapult me into a whole new world of healing and advocacy that I never expected to be a part of. I committed to learning as much as I could about alternative methods for healing, and this plunge into inquiry ultimately led me to cannabis and medicinal mushrooms as the all-star players of his healing team. To get there, I had to sift through a lot of conflicting information and red tape, due to the ever-changing legality of cannabis—and although the majority of medicinal mushrooms are legal, their powers are still largely unknown by many people. I gathered as much information as possible, from as many sources and studies as I could find, and I moved home to my parents' town for a few months so I could take on the most important role I've ever stepped into—the role of my dad's health coach.

This is how I unexpectedly became passionate about two classifications of plant medicine commonly thought of as "drugs." The information I found was astounding—not only are there countless stories of cannabis and mushrooms helping people with serious conditions like cancer, but I learned that these plants and fungi have been used as medicines for healing and wellness for thousands of years.

Under my guidance (and with his oncologist's blessing), my dad began to add cannabis and medicinal mushrooms into his daily routine alongside his chemotherapy treatments. Shortly after starting on that regimen, he started to feel better—the side effects he was initially experiencing from the chemotherapy lifted. Since then, he's been able to avoid all of the most common (and often debilitating) side effects of chemo. He has no nausea, his appetite is great, his mood is positive, his energy is high, and his immune system is strong. His tumors have remained stable and dormant for two years since his diagnosis, and his tumor blood markers are back down in the normal range and continue to improve. His doctors say his progress is "remarkable."

My dad's quality of life has been, in many ways, better than it was before he had cancer—he's been traveling, playing golf, and feeling great most of the time. While we can't say with absolute certainty it's the cannabis and mushrooms that are causing him to feel so good, we definitely believe they've played a major role in enhancing his quality of life. Most important, we've been able to spend an incredible amount of time together as we embarked on this adventure of learning, healing, and progress.

As I researched cannabis and mushrooms for improving my dad's quality of life during cancer treatment, I began to uncover a wealth of knowledge about using them for everyday wellness. I started experimenting with them myself—to help me sleep, to support my immune system when I was feeling under the weather, to calm my anxiety, to ease my menstrual cramps, to give me energy, and to help me focus on my work. Some of the effects were subtle; some were more profound. My own home became a "rebel's apothecary," as I started incorporating cannabis and mushrooms into my morning-to-evening routines.

I started recommending CBD and medicinal mushrooms to my friends. I posted about our experience on my blog and social media, and emails started pouring in with questions—not only from people who are interested in everyday wellness, but from people who are really struggling. Many of these messages come from caregivers just like me who have family members with cancer. In fact, we got so many messages that my dad and I created a guide to managing chemo side effects, which is included in this book.

I can feel the pain and uncertainty in every message I get, and I knew I needed to share this information in a clear, accessible way. Not with the intention to cure anything—but to help people take their quality of life into their own hands. *To help people feel better.*

The power of cannabis and mushrooms reaches far beyond just me and my dad. I continue to learn more about how cannabis and mushrooms are helping people every day. To do my research for this book, I've attended medicinal mushroom seminars and medical cannabis conferences, gone on mushroom-foraging walks, and learned directly from herbalists, mycologists, doctors, and scientists. The more I learn, the more fascinating cannabis and mushrooms become to me.

In the two years since I started sharing about these topics, many of the same people who were reaching out to me in a moment of hopelessness are now sharing messages of hope. These days, every time I open my inbox I find stories from people who have tried cannabis and medicinal mushrooms and found relief—from both everyday concerns and more serious conditions.

I'm not a doctor, and I'm not claiming to have the answers that will heal you. But my world has been completely illuminated by the research I've done on cannabis and mushrooms, and I believe they can offer us potent medicines if we learn how to work with them. My intention is to arm you with information to help you enhance your own life, whether you want to feel better during chemotherapy or just finally get a good night's sleep.

First, I'll teach you all about cannabis and why our bodies are so nourished by it. We'll go over CBD, THC, and how to use cannabis without feeling intoxicated (now that you know my story, you know I care a lot about that aspect).

After that, I'll guide you through the wild world of mushrooms, and you'll meet some of the most potent medicinal mushrooms in the fungi kingdom.

Once you get acquainted with cannabis and mushrooms, I'll guide you through protocols for daily wellness and share a few delicious cannabis- and mushroom-infused recipes so you can easily incorporate them into your life. In this section, you'll find help with reducing pain, alleviating anxiety, improving your mood, enhancing your energy, sleeping more deeply, and more.

From there, we'll move on to learn about cannabis, mushrooms, and cancer—and how to help manage chemotherapy side effects if you're going through treatment.

As you make your way through this book, I'll help you clear any confusion you may have, so you can create your own "rebel's apothecary"—stocked with exactly what you need to start feeling better. (We'll even cover magic mushrooms, and I'll share some of the latest research with you!)

You'll notice that I mention some specific brands throughout the book and in the Resources section, as these are the brands I trust, have experienced benefits from, and enjoy using at the time of this writing. To see an updated list, head to RebelsApothecary.com/Resources.

You can read through this whole book start to finish, or simply flip to the section that addresses what you want help with in this moment. It's here for you anytime you need a guide along your healing path.

As I write this, I'm sitting in my parents' kitchen. My dad is outside doing work in the yard, enjoying the fruits of his tomato and cucumber garden (he says planting is a sign of optimism—that you'll be around to enjoy the harvest). He's still going through chemo treatments, and he's still using cannabis and mushrooms every day. Two years after one of the darkest days of his life, my dad's motto is: "If I didn't know I was sick, I wouldn't know I was sick!" He smiles and laughs every single time he says it. Seeing that sparkle in his eye and knowing his suffering has been lifted—that is the greatest gift. You'll hear more about his story from him directly, on page 249.

As for me, I never thought I would put cannabis and mushrooms into my body on a daily basis, but they've become a fundamental part of my everyday life. My perception of them has completely changed, as I've learned to use them in quite a different way than I did in college—

without any intoxicating effects. They've found a home together in this book because the questions I get about them are always the same. When I mention CBD or cannabis, the first comment is often "But I don't want to get high," and when I mention medicinal mushrooms, I commonly hear, "Am I going to hallucinate?" Once you learn to use them without fear or uncertainty, they may quickly become a cherished part of your daily life, too.

As you begin to create your own "rebel's apothecary," I think you'll find cannabis and mushrooms just as enchanting as I do. I hope the information in this book sends you on a great journey of healing, fascination, and well-being—and encourages you to form a relationship with plants, herbs, and mushrooms for the rest of your life.

Love,

Jenny Sansouci

PART 1
CANNABIS AND MUSHROOMS 101

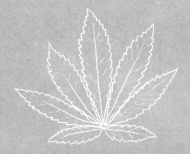

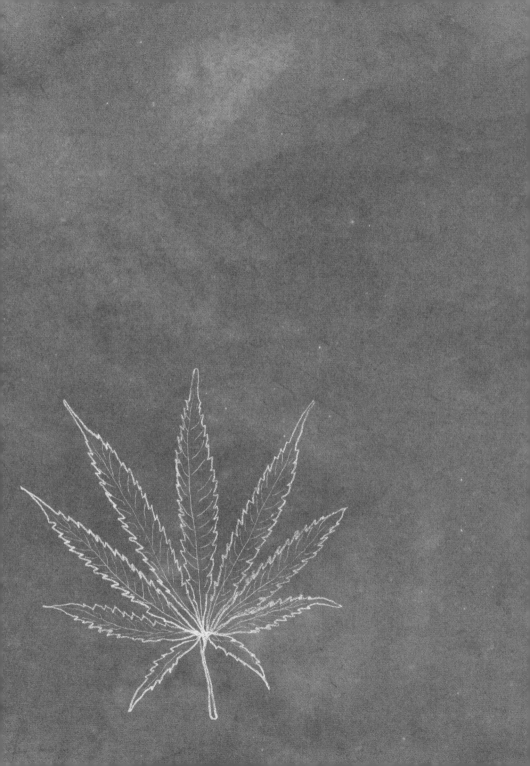

THE RENAISSANCE OF
CANNABIS AND MUSHROOMS

We are on the brink of one of the biggest cultural shifts in history. A major revolution is happening right now in drug policy and plant medicine—one that future generations will always look back on as historically significant . . . as the time when everything changed.

THE RENAISSANCE OF CANNABIS

For many people, there's still a great deal of resistance that comes along with accepting cannabis as a medicine. Because the cannabis plant has been categorized as an illicit drug for so long, the "reefer madness" stigma will take some time to lift completely. At the time of this writing, cannabis is a Schedule 1 controlled substance in the United States, which is defined as a drug that has a high potential for abuse and no accepted medical use. We know now that with cannabis, this is not the case. All anecdotal stories of healing aside, there are already accepted medical uses for cannabis in the pharmaceutical world, with at least four prescription drugs currently available that are derived from cannabis molecules. Legalization is shifting, and cannabis could soon become federally legal in the United States.

Cannabis has been used traditionally as a medicine for thousands of years, with many of the early cannabis plants traced back to Asia and India. Some of the earliest verified evidence of cannabis use by humans was more than 3,000 years ago in Egypt, and at least 2,500 years ago in China—where it was listed as one of the fifty fundamental herbs of traditional Chinese medicine.

Cannabis wasn't introduced to Western medicine until 1841, when an Irish physician named William O'Shaughnessy brought it over to Europe from India. From there, the medical use of cannabis spread to the United States, and in 1850 it was listed as a medicine in the *United States Pharmacopoeia*—an annually published collection of drug information. Doctors became familiar with recommending cannabis as a medicine for pain, insomnia, and depression. Throughout much of the 1800s, cannabis tinctures were sold in pharmacies and were a staple home remedy in medicine cabinets across the country.

In 1937, however, the first step toward total prohibition happened with the passage of the Marihuana Tax Act. This act administered a prohibitive tax on cannabis buyers, sellers, importers, growers, physicians, and anyone else in possession of it—and in 1942, cannabis was dropped from the *United States Pharmacopoeia* completely. The Controlled Substances Act of 1970 officially prohibited cannabis under federal law, as Harry Anslinger (the first commissioner of the Federal Bureau of Narcotics) spearheaded the decades-long failure that was the War on Drugs. The War on Drugs led to mass incarceration—disproportionately targeting communities of color and criminalizing people for mere possession of the "dangerous drug" they called "marijuana"—even though there had never been any evidence that it caused harm.

> By getting the public to associate the hippies with marijuana and blacks with heroin, and then criminalizing both heavily, we could disrupt those communities. We could arrest their leaders, raid their homes, break up their meetings, and vilify them night after night on the evening news.
>
> —John Ehrlichman, counsel and assistant to the president for domestic affairs under Richard Nixon, in a 1994 interview with Dan Baum published in 2016 in Harper's Magazine

Another great tragedy of the War on Drugs is the fact that so many people were denied the medicine they needed at the time they needed it most. This is still happening today. Much of the fight to legalize cannabis throughout the past few decades has been focused on getting medicine to patients—cancer patients, AIDS patients, epilepsy patients, and people using cannabis to alleviate pain and have a better quality of life. Even in cases where it was clear that this plant was helping, it was often seized or confiscated, and patients were denied access to the medicine that could help them to survive. The unnecessary suffering caused by the War on Drugs is only beginning to be alleviated, which could give way to a new era of humans having the freedom to use cannabis therapeutically, without fear of persecution.

Even now, with so many strides toward legalization in the United States, and CBD recently becoming federally legal, the "reefer madness" mindset is still alive, and the cannabis plant is still considered a Schedule 1 drug, right up there with heroin.

The Schedule 1 classification controls how much research can legally be done, which hinders the kind of studies we need to truly understand the plant's therapeutic benefits. But the fact that we can walk into a store and buy CBD oil, and that many of us can now walk into a dispensary and purchase medical cannabis or grow our own plants— it's a huge step forward.

Because CBD has been shown (in both scientific research and anecdotally) to have so many medical benefits, and no intoxicating effects, it can no longer be ignored.

"Societal attitudes toward cannabis have changed considerably in recent years, and the huge popularity of CBD has been a big factor," says Martin A. Lee, director of Project CBD and author of *Smoke Signals: A Social History of Marijuana—Medical, Recreational, and Scientific*. "The cat's out of the bag," he says. "You can't put the genie back in the bottle." CBD's therapeutic benefits have helped to destigmatize THC, and the whole cannabis plant for that matter, and restore its reputation as an important medicinal herb.

It's a privilege to be able to enjoy using cannabis today for wellness and health without legal consequences, and to speak about it as a medicine. While we learn to use cannabis therapeutically in our everyday lives, we can't forget about the fight that has been going on and the injustices that have occurred to get us where we are today. Advocacy for cannabis as medicine goes hand in hand with advocacy for prisoners with unjust marijuana convictions—that they will continue to be released, their criminal records expunged, and that they can get the support they need to enter the cannabis industry legally (if they want to), or otherwise have support in reentering their communities. Some of these changes are already under way or are being promised by prospective political candidates. The world of cannabis is changing, and we're on the forefront of those shifts now. To stay up to date on how you can support cannabis reform legislation, head to the Resources section.

THE RISE OF MEDICINAL MUSHROOMS

Thankfully, most of the medicinal mushrooms I'll cover in this book have never been illegal or controlled. Medicinal mushrooms have been used in traditional Chinese medicine for centuries, and their use is becoming more and more widespread in Western society as we become aware of their health benefits. We'll cover seven different species of mushrooms in *The Rebel's Apothecary*, but the only mushrooms we'll touch upon together that have been outlawed are the psychedelic mushrooms—you may know them as "magic mushrooms," and they contain a psychedelic compound called psilocybin. Psilocybin is also currently a Schedule 1 controlled substance in the United States, although it's been decriminalized in cities like Denver and Oakland, with more on the horizon. Psilocybin is being studied for use in therapy for treatment-resistant depression as we speak, with many potential developments still to come.

Psychedelic mushrooms are experiencing their own renaissance. These mushrooms were just beginning to be researched in the 1960s, when they, like cannabis, got hit with a Schedule 1 drug classification in 1970, which halted research. As research has been revving back up, it's predicted that psilocybin will be legally available for patients in therapeutic settings within the next few years.

Along with the rise, reacceptance, and decriminalization of magic mushrooms, the use of non-psychedelic medicinal mushrooms has been gaining more and more popularity. Medicinal mushrooms are being crowned in the wellness world as "superfoods," as they're popping up in coffee shops and being added to smoothies all over the country. These mushrooms have become welcome additions to everyday wellness routines, and their benefits are quickly becoming mainstream. And with good reason—all of these mushrooms have ancient histories as medicines, just like cannabis.

As cannabis legalization becomes widespread and mushrooms rise to stardom, I hope this book will drop into your hands at the perfect time and illuminate the path ahead for you. I hope you'll come away from this book with an understanding of how to safely and effectively use cannabis therapeutics and medicinal mushrooms to upgrade your quality of life and expand your field of vision about what's possible.

Cannabis and mushrooms are staged to become some of the most groundbreaking plant medicines for human health. Let's get to know them now.

LET'S TALK ABOUT CANNABIS

DEMYSTIFYING THE CANNABIS PLANT

Cannabis is finally having its day in the sun—or at least peeking its head out into the sun. As the doors open up for us to enjoy a legal relationship with this medicinal plant, we're truly only beginning to understand its vast array of healing benefits. Once legalization shifts and proper human clinical trials with cannabis can get under way, a whole new world will open up for so many who need it.

For now, let's get acquainted with the cannabis plant. Once you understand the medicine that's inside the plant, you'll be well on your way to using it safely—as a healing ally.

HEMP VS. MARIJUANA

Hemp, cannabis, marijuana—you've probably heard many different terms thrown around in the wild world of cannabis, and it can be confusing to figure out what's what. Cannabis is a plant in the botanical family *Cannabaceae,* which encompasses what we think of as the "hemp" plant as well as what we think of as the "marijuana" plant. Hemp and marijuana are both cannabis plants. As it legally stands today, the only thing separating "hemp" from "marijuana" is the amount of delta-9-tetrahydrocannabinol (or THC) in it—that's the part of the plant that gets you high.

As of now in the United States, "hemp" is legally considered a variety of the cannabis plant with a THC content of .3 percent or less. "Marijuana" is legally considered a variety of the cannabis plant that contains *more* than .3 percent THC. Any cannabis product with a THC level higher than .3 percent is currently only legal at licensed dispensaries, but not legal to purchase in stores or online. Cannabis plants are now being bred to have many different percentages of THC in them to address specific customer and patient needs, but they can only be legally purchased at dispensaries.

CBD (*cannabidiol*), the wildly popular, non-intoxicating compound in the cannabis plant, has gained its own legal traction as of late, but the details as to what's legal and what's not can be challenging to navigate. At the time of this writing, CBD products with .3 percent THC content or less are considered to be from hemp and are federally legal in the United States as of 2018. Any CBD product that goes over that .3 percent THC limit is legal only in states that have licensed medical or adult-use dispensaries. The .3 percent is an arbitrary number, however, and the FDA is currently working on more specific regulations and guidelines for CBD products. If cannabis becomes federally legal in the United States, the .3 percent number would become obsolete.

Because "cannabis" is the botanical name for these plants, it's the one we're going to use, and it's the one most experts and scientists use, instead of marijuana (which is a term that surfaced during the War on Drugs, and was used in racial propaganda against the plant by associating the word with Mexican immigrants). The term "marijuana" is still used today because it's currently the way the law distinguishes between the different levels of THC in cannabis plants (and therefore what's legal to sell in different states).

MALE AND FEMALE CANNABIS PLANTS

"When it comes to making CBD oil," says Martin A. Lee, "it's all about the amount of resin the plant produces. That's where the medicine is." This sticky resin comes out of "trichomes" on the cannabis flower, which look like tiny little straws with liquid bursting out of their tops.

There are two sexes of cannabis—male and female. Technically, hermaphrodite plants can grow, too—these plants have both male pollen sacs and female flowers.

The large flowers (or "buds") and the resin needed to produce CBD oil and all other forms of cannabis medicine come from the female cannabis plant only. The male plants produce the pollen that pollinates females to create new seeds, but males don't produce the flowers themselves. The males are useful in the case of industrial hemp fibers (to make things such as clothing, rope, and textiles) but not for medicine.

Many cannabis growers focus on growing female plants only, and clone their female plants in order to be sure their crop is all female. The crops have to be checked on a regular basis, and if a male pops up, it is usually removed immediately so it doesn't pollinate the females. If pollinated, the females will focus most of their energy on producing seeds rather than the coveted buds. Therefore, the male plants have to be separated and discarded, so the unfertilized females can have the space to grow and bloom to their fullest potential.

I recently went to visit a hemp farm in Maine that grows cannabis for CBD oil. There were rows and rows of beautiful hemp plants covering the rolling hills of the farm, which the grower said he has to walk through constantly, checking for rogue males that could potentially pollinate the whole crop. He was even worried about the pollen from male plants on neighboring farms, traveling in on the wind and making its way over to his females. It's a common fear among cannabis growers, since the females need to remain completely untouched by

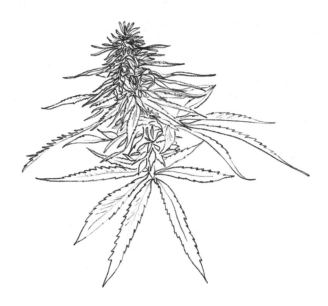

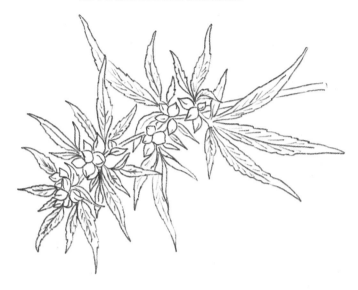

males to grow their big, resinous, medicinal buds. If you were start-ing to feel bad for the males, don't worry. There *is* a time when having male cannabis plants around is helpful—especially when growers want to produce a new strain of cannabis by breeding two strains together. Once this happens, the female cannabis plant will produce seeds that can be planted to grow new cannabis plants, which will have a fifty-fifty chance of being male or female.

Discovering whether your cannabis plant is male or female is called sexing the plant, and it's generally pretty easy to tell once the plant is about four to six weeks old. You can easily tell a male from a female cannabis plant once they start to reach maturity, because the males will grow pollen sacs, whereas the female plants will sprout tiny white hairs called "stigma," and then they will begin to produce large buds with sticky resin. Sexing the plant is all about what grows in between the "nodes" of the stems: If you see pollen sacs, it's a male. If you see little white hairs forming, it's female.

THE MEDICINE INSIDE THE CANNABIS PLANT

The reason these cannabis buds are so precious to us is because of the *hundreds* of active chemical compounds within the cannabis plant that we can use for medicine. These compounds include cannabinoids, terpenes, and flavonoids, and all of them work together to provide us with the medicinal benefits that are still being discovered on a daily basis.

THC and CBD are both cannabinoids, and are the most prevalent and well-known compounds in the cannabis plant. Even if you're a total cannabis newbie, you've probably heard of them. And if you haven't, well, sit down, grab a cup of tea, and let me be the first to acquaint you.

THC

THC is short for delta-9-tetrahydrocannabinol, and it's the psychoactive compound inside the cannabis plant that makes you feel the "high."

Although THC is famous for its intoxicating effects, it's also known for having a deep reservoir of healing benefits. A few of the most widely reported benefits include relief from pain and nausea, mood enhancement, and reducing inflammation—and it's even been shown to have antitumor properties.

Although cannabis has been used for its medicinal qualities for centuries, it wasn't until 1964 that a team of researchers in Israel, led by Professor Raphael Mechoulam at the Hebrew University of Jerusalem, isolated and described THC's molecular properties in a lab. Mechoulam is known as the father of cannabis medicine, as his team has made many advances in the field—including key contributions to the discovery of the system in the human body that cannabis works with to deliver its therapeutic benefits, which we'll cover in a minute.

While doing research for this book, I had the opportunity to hear Professor Mechoulam speak at the annual CannMed conference in Los Angeles (which was exciting, after spending so much time reading about his discoveries). He spoke about his work with cannabis compounds in his laboratory, and said the cannabis plant has been shown to be helpful for so many conditions—including depression, anxiety, epilepsy, cancer, schizophrenia, pain, inflammation, addiction, post-traumatic stress disorder (PTSD), autism, and autoimmune disease. He emphasized that the compounds in cannabis are not toxic to humans, and it's only because of the current legal situation that we are not able to do research that would potentially help millions of people who are suffering.

"We know that cannabis has anticancer activity, and we know that cancer patients who take cannabinoids live longer. This has been shown," he said. "We need clinical trials." However, the Schedule 1 classification of cannabis limits the amount of research that can be done.

CBD

"Yes, CBD is a fad right now—but there's something underneath the fad that should not be dismissed. CBD is a powerful molecule," says Martin A. Lee.

You can't walk down the street these days without seeing CBD. Short for cannabidiol, this compound is the wellness world's current darling. CBD is THC's non-psychoactive sister molecule, and it's another one of the most prevalent compounds inside the cannabis plant. Because it's just become federally legal in the United States, it's absolutely everywhere—and currently unregulated, which makes it challenging (but not impossible) to safely navigate products. CBD won't make you feel high—but it does have an incredible number of therapeutic effects—including soothing pain, anxiety, and inflammation.

The powers of CBD are just beginning to be embraced by the masses, with much more research to come in the future as legality continues to shift and more regulations are put in place. Because the medical benefits of CBD are becoming so widely known, the whole cannabis plant is getting closer and closer to federal legalization every day.

Three of the most common types of cannabis plants:

Type 1: high levels of THC

Type 2: a more or less equal combination
of CBD and THC

Type 3: high levels of CBD

Each cannabis type has different potential benefits, depending on the condition and the dose, and different "strains" (or chemical varieties) of cannabis have varying amounts of each compound. Some varieties of cannabis are bred to have higher levels of THC, and some (especially because of the CBD boom that's happening currently) are bred to have higher levels of CBD. The levels of THC and CBD present in each variety will have a different effect on your body and mind.

HEMP SEED OIL VS. CBD OIL

If you see a bottle labeled "hemp seed oil," it's not the same thing as CBD oil—they come from completely different parts of the plant.

Hemp seeds, hemp seed oil, and hemp milk (made from hemp seeds) are all rich in nutrients and fatty acids and great for adding to food and skincare, but they don't contain CBD or THC.

The seeds and stalk of the hemp plant are the parts used for food, fiber, and clothing—and as we learned before, the CBD and THC are found in the flower.

CBD LOWERS THC'S INTOXICATING EFFECTS

Higher levels of THC can be more therapeutic for some people, depending on their condition, but the more THC in the product, the greater the chance of feeling psychoactive effects. For some, this feeling is welcome and enjoyed; for others, it's unwanted. If CBD is present in the cannabis strain in high enough amounts, it can safeguard you from the psychoactive effects of THC. That's because CBD swoops in and partially blocks the THC from binding effectively to receptors in the brain. **The higher the CBD-to-THC ratio in a cannabis product, the less likely you are to feel a high.**

THE ENTOURAGE EFFECT

There were never so many able, active minds at work on the problems of diseases as now, and all their discoveries are tending to the simple truth—that you can't improve on nature.
—*Thomas Edison, 1903*

CBD is paving the way for the rest of the cannabis plant to be legalized, and one of the reasons is that the compounds in the cannabis plant have been shown to work better together (as a whole-plant extract), rather than as separate compounds in isolation.

THC and CBD may be the stars of the show when it comes to the cannabinoids, but there are hundreds of active compounds (cannabinoids, terpenes, and flavonoids) in the cannabis plant, and all of them work together to make it the healing powerhouse that it is.

These compounds work together to produce stronger medicinal effects than when isolated—this is called the entourage effect.

The entourage effect is the reason getting "full-spectrum" or "whole-plant extract" matters when it comes to the medicinal and health-enhancing effects of cannabis. The molecules within the plant complement one another's strengths—they boost each other up.

Dr. Annemarie Colbin, founder of the Natural Gourmet Institute in New York City and author of *Food and Healing,* was one of my most treasured nutrition teachers. One of the things I'll always remember from my time studying with her was her viewpoint on eating "whole foods" vs. "fragmented foods." She described whole foods as "those that nature provides, with all their edible parts." Fragmented foods, on the other hand, are missing some of their original parts (for example, processed foods that have ingredients that are isolated from the original food source).

"We are programmed to survive on what the Earth provides," said Dr. Colbin. "When you eat a fragmented food, your body is out of balance, searching for the rest of it."

We can think about cannabis in the same way. Of course, there can be some benefits from the use of isolated molecules from the cannabis plant (in pharmaceutical form or otherwise), but it has been shown that the whole-plant extracts can have a more significant effect than a single molecule alone—and often, a lower dose is needed when the full spectrum of plant compounds are taken together.

As Dr. Ethan Russo, a prominent cannabis researcher and board-certified neurologist, notes in his 2019 paper "The Case for the Entourage Effect and Conventional Breeding of Clinical Cannabis," when it comes to the pharmaceutical CBD drug Epidiolex (a 97 percent pure CBD isolate, with THC removed, used to treat seizures), a much higher dose is necessary to achieve positive results (reduction in seizure frequency) than when using a CBD-rich full-spectrum cannabis extract with all the other compounds of the plant intact. When taking eleven different studies into account, results show that 71 percent of epilepsy patients improved with CBD-dominant, whole-plant cannabis extracts, vs. 36 percent improvement for the patients taking purified CBD isolate. "These studies and others provide a firm foundation for cannabis synergy, and support for botanical drug development vs. that of single components," says Russo.

CANNABIS STRAINS

All you have to do is walk into a dispensary to see the dizzying array of cannabis strains (or chemical varieties) available to you. Cannabis strains typically have playful names like Blue Dream, Strawberry Cough, and Super Silver Haze—but as tempting as it might be, there are better ways to pick your medicine than by the name alone. Each strain will have a different makeup of chemical compounds, each compound providing unique effects on the body and mind. Strains of cannabis are often bred together to combine their chemical profiles and produce the exact effects the grower or patient is looking for, which will lead to even more highly specified varieties of cannabis medicine in the future.

Some of the main factors that contribute to differences in cannabis strains:

- THC content

- CBD content

- Level of other cannabinoids and terpenes present

- The environment the cannabis plant was grown in (outdoor, sun-grown cannabis in California can produce different compounds and effects than indoor, greenhouse-grown cannabis in Vermont, for example—even if they have the same strain name).

Over the past few decades, most strains of cannabis have been bred to produce high levels of THC, for recreational use, as these strains were in the highest demand. This type of high-THC-only breeding is starting to shift as more people become interested in the benefits of using CBD and some of the other cannabinoids. There's a growing market of widespread demand for cannabis medicine that doesn't cause intoxicating effects. The future of cannabis strains is colorful, to say the least, as the possibilities for personalized cannabis medicine are nearly endless.

SATIVA AND INDICA

When cannabis was first discovered, plants from different regions in the world looked different physically. The cannabis varieties from India often had short, stubby, thick leaves (commonly referred to as "indica" plants) and the plants from Europe and Asia had long, thin, pointy leaves (commonly referred to as "sativa" plants). In the beginning of cannabis cultivation, these physical distinctions were more relevant, but at this point, the plants have been bred together so many times that many so-called sativa and indica strains look close to identical.

The terms "sativa" and "indica" are still used to describe the effects of the different cannabis strains, but today these terms are based on the chemical compounds inside the plant rather than the shape of the leaves.

Most people associate "indica" strains with a mellow, sedating, relaxing body high (and therefore good for evening use), and "sativa" strains with uplifting, elevating, and energizing effects (and therefore good for the daytime).

While "indica" and "sativa" can give you a direction for understanding a strain's effects, looking at the overall chemical profile can make more of a difference when understanding how it will make you feel. In fact, some cannabis doctors and scientists dissuade people from using the "sativa" and "indica" terms entirely. Once you become familiar with all of the different compounds within the cannabis plant and what they each do (coming up next!), you won't have to ask "Which one works better for sleep?" or "Which one is more uplifting?" You'll be able to decipher it on your own, which is an exciting and powerful thing.

Let's take a look at how cannabis works in the body and dive deeper into the entourage of characters inside the cannabis plant, so you can feel as informed as possible about what you need when you walk into a dispensary or when you order your CBD oil online.

> **IMPORTANT TIP TO REMEMBER**: No matter what the label says or which compounds are present in the cannabis product you choose, your personal experience is what will guide you. Try it, and see how you feel. It's very likely that you'll end up choosing different varieties, doses, and methods of delivery for different reasons, and cycle through them at different times, depending on your needs and desires.

Clinical cannabis has become a therapeutic compass
to what modern medicine fails to cure.
—*Dr. Ethan Russo*

THE ENDOCANNABINOID SYSTEM

One of the most fascinating things about using cannabis as medicine is that our bodies are actually designed to receive it. We have an entire regulatory system in the body with specific receptors that interact with the cannabinoids in the cannabis plant. It's called the endocannabinoid system (or ECS), and it's responsible for maintaining homeostasis, or balance, in virtually every system in the body. Learning how the endocannabinoid system works allows us to see exactly *why* cannabis can help us with so many things. From anxiety to immune support to mood to inflammation—the ECS regulates it all, and it plays a key role in keeping our health in balance.

In 1992, Professor Raphael Mechoulam and his team in Israel identified the first endocannabinoid molecule, which led to the discovery of the endocannabinoid system. The discovery of the endocannabinoid

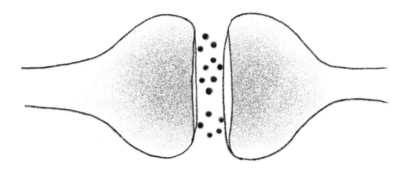

system originally stemmed from researchers working to determine exactly how THC works in the body. When they observed where the THC molecule traveled, they found receptors all throughout the body that interact with the compounds found in the cannabis plant.

There are three main parts to our endocannabinoid system (ECS):

- Endocannabinoid molecules
- Cannabinoid receptors
- Enzymes and proteins that create, break down, and transport endocannabinoids to our receptors

OUR NATURAL, INNER CANNABINOIDS

Although our endocannabinoid system interacts with the molecules inside the cannabis plant, the system doesn't exist in our bodies for cannabis alone. We produce our *own* cannabinoids naturally, and the cannabinoids from cannabis (like THC and CBD) interact with the same receptors. You can think of a receptor as a "lock" and cannabinoids as "keys." When a cannabinoid interacts with a receptor, a biochemical signal is sent to the body and we experience a physiological response (such as reduction in pain or anxiety).

The cannabinoids we make internally are called endocannabinoids ("endo" means "internal, or within"), and the cannabinoids we get from plants are called phytocannabinoids ("phyto" means "plant").

Our endocannabinoids help to regulate mood, stress, anxiety, pain, sleep, appetite, inflammation, memory, and the immune system. There are cannabinoid receptors located almost everywhere throughout the body, and when we fall out of balance in any of these areas, endocannabinoids are produced as needed to help us get back into balance. Our natural endocannabinoid levels go up in response to stress, pain, anxiety, and inflammation—and they can even prevent the retrieval of harmful memories, which points us to why some PTSD patients report relief from their symptoms when using cannabis.

ENDOCANNABINOIDS

Two of the main endocannabinoids that have been identified so far are called anandamide and 2-AG.

Anandamide. Anandamide was named after the Sanskrit word for bliss, *"ananda,"* and is often referred to as the "bliss molecule." This endocannabinoid has been shown to be involved in mood enhancement and a decrease in depression and anxiety. It's associated with giving us the "runner's high" (often experienced as euphoria and lessened perception of pain) experienced after a workout. Hence, the nickname "bliss molecule."

2-AG. 2-AG is the most abundant endocannabinoid found in the body, and it plays an important role in the regulation of appetite, the immune system, and pain management. To top it off, a 2017 study published in *The Journal of Sexual Medicine* found that 2-AG is greatly increased during orgasm. (Why 2-AG wasn't coined the "bliss molecule," we shall never know.)

According to Professor Mechoulam, depression has been linked to low anandamide levels, and anxiety has been linked to low levels of 2-AG. "It's quite frankly outrageous that anandamide and 2-AG have not yet been directly administered to humans," says Mechoulam.

When we use cannabis, the compounds from the cannabis plant directly affect our natural endocannabinoid levels. THC binds directly to our cannabinoid receptors and mimics the effects of our endocannabinoids, while CBD works with our endocannabinoid system not by binding to the receptors but by blocking the enzymes that break down our natural endocannabinoids. CBD "upregulates" our endocannabinoid system—therefore, when we consume a CBD-rich cannabis product, we'll have higher levels of endocannabinoids circulating through our body, which can help alleviate a variety of ailments.

According to Dr. Ethan Russo, we all have a different baseline "endocannabinoid tone," which refers to the abundance and state of our endocannabinoids and receptors. Our diet, lifestyle, and genetics can have an effect on our endocannabinoid tone, so no two endocannabinoid systems are exactly alike. In addition to having different baseline levels of endocannabinoids in our bodies, we each have enzymes that break down these endocannabinoids at different rates. This is why we each respond differently to the various methods of delivery and dosages of cannabis medicine, and why (as you'll learn soon) there isn't a "one-size-fits-all" protocol when it comes to cannabis dosing. It will probably take some experimenting to know how your endocannabinoid system responds best to cannabis. In the future, as the endocannabinoid system is studied in more depth, we'll likely have greater insight into testing our baseline endocannabinoid tone—which would help us become much more efficient in our cannabis dosing strategies.

"If we can measure endocannabinoid levels, we can help patients start at a more appropriate dose of cannabis medicine," says Dr. Bonni Goldstein, a cannabis doctor with a Los Angeles–based practice.

OUR CANNABINOID RECEPTORS

How can one plant possibly have so many therapeutic effects? The answer lies in the fact that there are cannabinoid receptors all throughout the human body, regulating everything from mood, to memory, to pain. There are at least two kinds of cannabinoid receptors that make up our endocannabinoid system—these are called CB1 receptors and CB2 receptors.

CB1 receptors are primarily located in the brain, spinal cord, and central nervous system. The CB1 receptors are often referred to as the "psychoactive receptors," as it's these receptors that are responsible for the intoxicating effects of cannabis—along with the mood-boosting and antianxiety effects. Our CB1 receptors also help to regulate pain, emotion, memory, movement, nausea, appetite, seizures, and digestion.

CB2 receptors are located primarily in the immune system, in the peripheral nervous system, and in many other organs in the body, in-

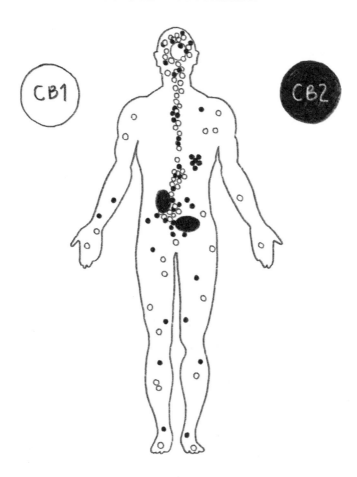

cluding the spleen, pancreas, and skin. CB2 receptors are often called the protective receptors, as they're responsible for regulating inflammation, immunity, and pain.

An example of the way CBD works with the endocannabinoid system is by inhibiting an enzyme called fatty acid amide hydrolase (FAAH), which breaks down anandamide (the "bliss molecule"). This leads to higher amounts of anandamide circulating in the body, which helps to explain some of CBD's mood-boosting and antianxiety effects. In this way, CBD enhances the body's natural endocannabinoid system without directly binding to the receptors.

Nourishing our endocannabinoid system can keep us feeling happy, healthy, and in balance—and cannabis can help support it in so many ways.

Aside from interacting with our CB1 and CB2 receptors, the medicinal molecules in cannabis interact with other receptors throughout the body—including TRPV1, which regulates pain; 5-HT1A, a serotonin receptor that regulates mood and anxiety; and GPR55, which plays a role in fighting cancer.

Did you know there have been zero reported deaths from cannabis overdose . . . ever? That's in sharp contrast to opioid overdose, which is the cause of more than 130 deaths per day in the United States, according to the National Institutes of Health (NIH) in 2019. There are very few cannabinoid receptors in the part of the brain that controls breathing and heart rate, so consuming too much cannabis won't lead to respiratory arrest—unlike opioids. Many people have reported lowering their opioid dose or getting off of opioids and other pain medications completely after starting a cannabis regimen for pain relief.

THE MINOR PHYTOCANNABINOIDS

CBD and THC are the most abundant phytocannabinoids inside the cannabis plant, but there's an entourage of "minor" cannabinoids contributing to the healing benefits of cannabis. The research on most of these cannabinoids is still in its infancy. Even though these minor cannabinoids are typically present in much lower amounts in most cannabis varieties, they each play a role in the overall entourage effect. Just as background actors are important to the overall effect of a movie scene, the tiniest amount of a minor cannabinoid can boost the strength and power of the others.

A few of the most prevalent minor cannabinoids are:

- **Cannabigerol (CBG).** Usually found in low amounts in most cannabis strains, CBG is known to be antibacterial, anti-inflammatory, and neuroprotective.

- **Cannabinol (CBN).** CBN is a breakdown product of THC, which means there is typically little to no CBN in a freshly harvested cannabis plant. CBN only shows up when the cannabis gets older and THC degrades. CBN is thought to be sedating, and in the future we may see more cannabis products geared toward sleep that contain higher levels of CBN.

- **Cannabichromene (CBC).** CBC is known to relieve pain and reduce inflammation, and has antibacterial properties. Like CBD, it can also inhibit the breakdown of anandamide (the bliss molecule), leading to elevation in mood and reduction in anxiety.

- **Cannabidiolic acid (CBDA).** CBDA is present in raw cannabis, and when heated it converts to CBD. CBDA in raw cannabis has been shown to have anti-inflammatory, antinausea, antianxiety, and anticancer effects, even before it's converted into CBD. Cannabis scientists are currently beginning to take a look at the potential therapeutic value of CBDA.

- **Tetrahydrocannabinolic acid (THCA).** Just like CBDA, THCA is an acid cannabinoid that's present in raw cannabis before it's heated. Once heated, it's converted into THC. THCA has been shown to be largely non-intoxicating and has anti-inflammatory and antinausea properties, so consuming cannabis products that haven't been exposed to heat may have some potent health benefits.

TERPENES

Terpenes, nicknamed "terps," are the aromatic compounds found in cannabis, as well as many other plants. The terpenes in cannabis not only give each strain a different scent, but they contribute to how the cannabis will make you feel.

One of the reasons you'll see people smelling the different cannabis flowers at a dispensary is because the scent says something about the individual terpene profile. Some say the scent you're most attracted to is the one your body needs the most at that time. While I can't prove this, I really like that idea. It's like when you gravitate to or crave different vegetables or nutrients at different times, they might be something your body needs, nutritionally. With this in mind, it can be interesting to notice which scents you're most attracted to when you visit a dispensary.

Here's a list of a few of the top terpenes you'll find in cannabis. This list is by no means exhaustive, as there are hundreds of terpenes— cannabis really does have a *huge* entourage. Not all cannabis products have the terpene profiles listed on them, but the market is headed that way. When you do find yourself in the presence of an array of cannabis options with different terpenes listed, you're in for a treat. This is when you can really have fun and get personalized about your cannabis medicine.

Some of the top terpenes are:

- **Limonene.** Limonene is a citrusy terpene that can produce uplifting, mood-elevating, and antidepressant effects—just like the scent of lemons or other citrus fruits. Limonene gives the smell and flavor to the more bright, citrusy strains of cannabis. If you're attracted to the mood-elevating effects of limonene, you'll likely enjoy the smell of a high-limonene strain. Strains of cannabis that are high in limonene are often associated with more of a "sativa" effect—uplifting and energizing, rather than sedating. Limonene is also known for helping mitigate the high from THC—so if you feel you've overconsumed THC, eating lemons or other citrus fruit or smelling citrus scents may help bring down the high. Outside of cannabis, limonene can be found in citrus rinds, rosemary, and peppermint.

- **Myrcene.** Myrcene is the most prevalent of all terpenes in cannabis, and it's the terpene to look for if you want a strain that will help you with sleep. In fact, the presence of myrcene is thought to be what actually dictates the indica vs. sativa effect! According to SC Labs, a cannabis testing company that does terpene analysis, cannabis strains containing .5 percent or more of myrcene produce an "indica" effect—which is more sedative, and can contribute to the sleepiness or "couch-lock" effect experienced with certain cannabis strains. If a strain has less than .5 percent myrcene, it can have a more "sativa" effect, energizing and uplifting. Myrcene's scent is often described as "earthy" and "herbal." Other plants containing myrcene include thyme, hops, and lemongrass.

- **Pinene.** Pinene has the piney scent of a forest, and is known to be the "focus" terpene. Like limonene, it can also counteract the fuzzy-memory effects of consuming too much THC. Strains high in pinene can be stimulating and alerting, and are known to be anti-inflammatory. Because pinene can help bring your mind back into focus if you've had too much THC, it's often recommended to sniff something pine scented (or eat pine nuts!) when you need to mitigate the effects of THC. In nature, pinene can also be found in sage, rosemary, frankincense, and—you guessed it—pine trees.

- **Caryophyllene.** Caryophyllene is a special terpene because it's the only terpene that's *also* a cannabinoid. That means it interacts with the body's endocannabinoid system directly—specifically, the CB2 receptors, which are located primarily in the immune system. Caryophyllene is known for its anti-inflammatory and pain-relieving effects, and can help with anxiety and depression. Caryophyllene has a spicy aroma and is also found in black pepper, cloves, copaiba, hops, and rosemary.

- **Linalool.** Linalool is a calming terpene with a floral scent; it's also found in lavender. Strains high in linalool can be great to help with stress and anxiety, just like you'd expect with lavender. Linalool is known for helping with relaxation and sleep, so if you find a strain of cannabis or cannabis product that has higher levels of linalool present, you can likely count on it to be a bit more relaxing. Aside from lavender, linalool can be found in basil, rose, cinnamon, and mint.

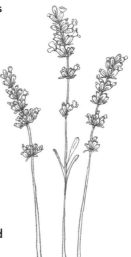

FLAVONOIDS

Flavonoids are naturally occurring pigments found in many plants, and are responsible for giving fruits, vegetables, flowers, and herbs their color and flavor. Truth be told, I cared way more about cannabinoids and terpenes than I did flavonoids while doing my research for this book, as flavonoids are the least-prevalent compounds in the cannabis plant (and the least studied, comparatively). But when a study recently came out showing that a flavonoid from cannabis could potentially be a treatment for pancreatic cancer, I paid attention. The molecule used in the study was a derivative of a cannabis flavonoid called cannaflavin B.

This finding further demonstrates the importance of the entourage effect—the presence of terpenes, cannabinoids, and flavonoids is an important reason to use "full-spectrum" or "whole-plant" extract when you're choosing a cannabis or CBD product—all of these compounds work synergistically to create a health-enhancing symphony. The whole is stronger than its parts, and each compound can add something unique and delightful to your wellness plan.

PHARMACEUTICAL CANNABIS PRODUCTS

Aside from endocannabinoids (produced naturally in the body) and phytocannabinoids (found in plants), there's a third type of cannabinoid that exists—the synthetic cannabinoid. This is the type of cannabinoid that's used in pharmaceutical drugs. When one cannabinoid is used on its own, away from the rest of the plant, it's called an isolate. Isolated molecules are the standard for how the majority of pharmaceutical drugs are studied, tested, and formulated. Although there can be benefits to isolated molecules, as they can easily be standardized, once you isolate one compound from the plant and put it by itself in a synthetic form, it's no longer considered "plant medicine," and the entourage effect no longer applies.

There are currently a few pharmaceutical products on the market made with cannabinoids (which require a prescription), but I expect many more to come as more cannabis research is conducted.

Examples of three pharmaceutical cannabis products that are available today:

- **Epidiolex: an isolated CBD-only pharmaceutical, prescribed to treat epileptic seizures**
- **Marinol: an isolated THC-only pharmaceutical, prescribed for chemotherapy-induced nausea and cancer pain**

- **Sativex:** a whole-plant extract with a 1:1 ratio of CBD to THC in a sublingual spray, prescribed for multiple sclerosis (MS) spasticity (Sativex is not approved in the United States at the time of this writing)

Synthetic, standardized molecules, although they do have a place in medicine, can potentially come with more side effects than using the whole plant, as the plant's synergistic compounds work together to bring balance to the body. If you read a study about negative side effects from cannabis medicine (or any plant-based medicine), check to see if it was from a single isolated molecule or an extract of the whole plant.

> Synthesized corporate concoctions will never make the whole plant obsolete. While cannabinoid designer drugs may indeed work wonders in the future (let's hope so), these synthetic products can never replace the widespread use of cost-effective, organically grown, backyard bud— with its pungent, antioxidant-rich mixture of cannabinoids, terpenes and flavonoids, which interact synergistically to produce a holistic, therapeutic effect that exceeds the capacity of single-molecule remedies. The plant's only drawback? It's against the law.
>
> —*Martin A. Lee*, Smoke Signals: A Social History of Marijuana—Medical, Recreational, and Scientific

LABELS AND LAB TESTS

CBD products are popping up on shelves everywhere, but right now the CBD market is highly unregulated. This means there aren't standards for what needs to be on the label. Typically, there isn't a whole lot of information on the product label about the other cannabinoids or terpenes present in the product. You can (and are encouraged to) always ask for an independent, third-party lab test when buying CBD to see what's actually in it. CBD products are often mislabeled and the contents are misrepresented, so a lab test can help you to verify what you're purchasing.

In a 2018 study by the Institute for Research on Cannabinoids, eighty-four different CBD products were analyzed—and 70 percent of the products didn't contain the amount of CBD they claimed on the label. When you're choosing a CBD product, asking for a lab test is the best way to really know what's in it. If the company you're purchasing from doesn't have a lab test or "certificate of analysis" available on their website, get in touch with them and ask for one. Your product should be tested for purity, quality, and strength, and the contents should match

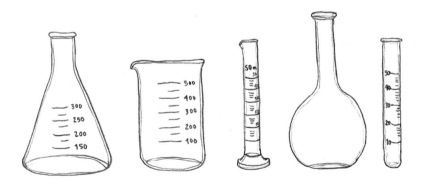

exactly what it says on the label. If a company refuses to provide a lab test, that's a red flag—don't buy it.

At the very least, the label on your cannabis or CBD product should tell you how many milligrams of CBD are in one serving of the product (for example, how many milligrams are in one milliliter if it's a tincture) and whether or not the product contains THC and, if so, how much.

If your CBD oil bottle doesn't give you the exact milligrams per milliliter, it should tell you the total amount of milligrams of CBD in the whole bottle. To calculate what you'll get in 1 ml (typically the amount in a dropperful of a tincture), take the total number of milligrams of CBD in the bottle and divide it by the total number of milliliters the bottle contains.

For example, if your bottle of CBD oil contains 1000 mg of CBD, and there are 30 ml in the bottle, each 1 ml dropperful will contain about 33 mg of CBD. You'd think all CBD oil labels would include this information, but because of the lack of label regulations, much of this sleuthing is ultimately left up to us.

It will soon become commonplace to personalize our cannabis and CBD preferences based on the full entourage, and as regulations shift we'll begin to see more details on product labels. As I learned when I took a tour of the CannaCraft cannabis oil production facility in Santa Rosa, California, each cannabinoid and terpene has a different molecular weight. This means laboratories are able to separate each compound out by weight, in order to determine exactly how much is present in a specific strain of cannabis, for accurate labeling and unique, personalized product formulations.

Cannabis consumers are becoming much more curious to understand exactly what's in each cannabis product, the same way we care about our food labels. This level of detail is something that is already happening in many licensed dispensaries, as they often have stricter regulations about lab testing and product quality than what you'd find at a health-food store or online.

These days, most reputable CBD companies will have lab tests available for consumers, either on the website or by request.

What to Look for on a Lab Test:

- The amount of CBD in the whole product, and the amount in each serving. Does the lab test match what the label claims?

- The amount of THC in the product, and in each serving

- The other cannabinoids and terpenes present (if this information is available). If a product's lab test offers terpene profiles, you know they are doing their groundwork.

- Verify that the product has tested negative for pesticides, heavy metals, and residual solvents. Cannabis is a bioaccumulator, meaning it absorbs whatever is in the soil, and certain extraction methods can leave residual solvents in the product—you want to make sure the cannabis product you're using is free of these chemicals. It will state this clearly on the lab test.

CBD OIL EXTRACTION

In order to extract the medicine from the cannabis plant, the plant goes through a multistep extraction process. The two most common extraction methods are supercritical CO_2 extraction and ethanol extraction. These methods remove the beneficial cannabinoids, terpenes, and flavonoids from the plant so they can be added into medicine. CO_2 extraction is considered to be one of the safest extraction methods, as well as one of the most common for commercial products. Ethanol extraction, on the other hand, is commonly used for some high-potency medical cannabis products (for example, Rick Simpson Oil [RSO] and Full Extract Cannabis Oil [FECO], which we'll cover in the cancer section). Extraction methods such as butane, hexane, and propane are considered less safe extraction methods, as these chemicals are neurotoxins and residual solvents can be left in the product. Regardless of which extraction method was used for the cannabis product you try, you'll want to check the lab test to make sure it tests negative for chemicals and solvents.

CBD: FULL-SPECTRUM, BROAD-SPECTRUM, ISOLATE

When you're looking for your first CBD product to try, it can be overwhelming to consider all of the options. One of the first things you'll notice is that CBD products are generally labeled:

- Full-spectrum or whole-plant
- Broad-spectrum
- Isolate

These three types of CBD products have different compositions, and may affect you differently, so it's important to pay attention to the details, and of course experiment for yourself to see how you feel.

I've experimented with all three, and I always choose full-spectrum because it seems to be the most powerful for sleep, pain, and anxiety. Many people have positive experiences with broad-spectrum and isolate products, too, so you don't have to rule them out as options—but in general, because of the entourage effect, many experts say the "fuller" the spectrum you can get, the better.

It's important to note these descriptive terms (full-spectrum, broad-spectrum, isolate, whole-plant) aren't regulated—so again, looking at a lab test is important if you really want to know what's in your product.

Full-Spectrum CBD

Full-spectrum CBD is typically considered a whole-plant extract. This means it should contain all components of the cannabis plant—the cannabinoids, terpenes, and flavonoids. A full-spectrum CBD product also usually includes some amount of THC—even if it's a tiny amount. Often, lower doses are required with a full-spectrum product, as the entourage effect is present to support the full power of the CBD.

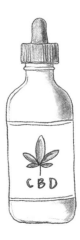

CBD Isolate

On the other end of the "spectrum" is CBD isolate, which is the CBD molecule only, with no other compounds from the plant present. People who choose a CBD isolate are often looking for a zero-THC product. You'll notice that when you consume a CBD isolate in oil form, it's often clear, odorless, and tasteless. While some may prefer this, as they don't like the "weed" taste of full-spectrum oil, you may find that you have to take a higher amount of isolate to find relief than you would with full-spectrum—since the entourage effect isn't working in your favor to boost the effects of the CBD. Just as removing a vitamin from a vegetable doesn't give you the full benefits of actually eating a vegetable, removing CBD from cannabis completely and isolating it doesn't provide the full benefits of consuming the whole plant.

Some companies hoping to capitalize on the CBD craze will take a small amount of full-spectrum CBD and add a huge amount of isolate on top of it, so they can claim to have a higher-milligram product but also still claim to be full-spectrum.

Recently, I bought a bottle of CBD isolate from a reputable company, and I tried it in the usual way I would use a full-spectrum oil (I took about 25 mg, in tincture form). I waited an hour, and I didn't feel any of the antianxiety or relaxing effects I generally do with full-spectrum oil. It may have worked better if I took it in larger amounts—many patients report needing about five times the amount of isolate to get the relief they would get with full-spectrum.

Broad-Spectrum CBD

A CBD product type that's fairly new on the scene is broad-spectrum CBD. Broad-spectrum is similar to full-spectrum, except the THC has been removed. It has the benefit of an isolate (no THC) but also the benefit of full-spectrum (other cannabinoids and terpenes are present to boost the power of the CBD). This means broad-spectrum CBD is likely to give you stronger effects than a CBD isolate, but potentially not as strong as full-spectrum. When I tried broad-spectrum, I was pleasantly surprised that I did experience the relaxing and calming effects of full-spectrum CBD, which I didn't feel with isolate. Broad-spectrum CBD could be a great option for daytime anxiety, or for people who want to avoid THC completely. I could also taste more of the plant in broad-spectrum oil than I did with the isolate product, which could be because the terpenes and flavonoids are still present.

THC'S PSYCHOACTIVE THRESHOLD

The psychoactive properties of THC are what cause the high from cannabis. Some people love the feeling; others want to avoid it completely. A high from THC can feel different to each individual, but the most commonly reported positive effects of THC include stress relief, euphoria, ease, heightened creativity, and enhanced enjoyment of activities. The most common negative effects include fatigue, impaired short-term memory, dry mouth, disorientation, fuzziness, brain fog, anxiety, and paranoia. Appetite stimulation is another common effect of THC (which could be considered positive or negative, depending on the circumstance).

The threshold for psychoactivity in sensitive users or people who don't use cannabis often is typically around 2 mg, but it's possible to feel the effects of THC at lower amounts. Personally, my body and mind react very sensitively to the slightest mood-altering substance— I can feel the effects of THC at about 1 mg.

For reference, a standard dose for THC products geared toward recreational use is typically about 5–10 mg—this will make most people feel high.

Different delivery methods will influence how THC makes you feel. So if you're comfortable experimenting, experiment. As they say, when trying any cannabis product: "Start low, and go slow." If you do experience any uncomfortable effects, take a note of how you felt and what amount you took, and take a smaller dose next time.

CHOOSING A CBD PRODUCT

When it comes to choosing a CBD product, the most important consideration is that you listen to your own body. What effects are you hoping to feel when taking the product? How important is the THC level to you?

If you're not worried about ingesting THC, I would definitely suggest trying out a full-spectrum product, so you'll get the full magic of cannabis as it's designed for your body's endocannabinoid system to receive. From there (if you have legal access to higher-THC products), you can experiment with different ratios of CBD and THC.

For some, the more THC present in a CBD product, the more the product works therapeutically. "Many people start out with a CBD isolate, then move to a full-spectrum CBD product, and eventually find relief with a CBD-rich product that has a little bit more THC than .3 percent," says Martin A. Lee.

THE CANNABIS AND CBD PRODUCTS YOU'LL FIND AT A DISPENSARY VS. ONLINE

If you're shopping for your CBD products at a health-food store or online, you'll typically find CBD products containing .3 percent THC or less. At licensed dispensaries, you'll find cannabis products with higher levels of THC than the federally legal .3 percent, and most dispensaries will offer many different CBD-to-THC ratio options. Many dispensaries have their menus available online, so you can check ahead of time to see if they have the product you're looking for.

MEDICAL VS. RECREATIONAL/ADULT-USE DISPENSARIES

As it stands today, out of the thirty-three states with legal medical cannabis, eleven also have legal recreational—or adult-use—laws. This means anyone over the age of twenty-one can legally purchase cannabis products at a dispensary. When describing dispensaries, "adult use" and "recreational" mean the same thing—but the term "adult use" is often preferred by cannabis users as a nod to the fact that so many people are using cannabis therapeutically, not solely for recreation.

Even in those states, however, some dispensaries are still medical only—meaning they provide cannabis only to patients with a doctor's recommendation. Typically, the patient must have a medical condition, qualify for a medical card, and get a doctor's approval to purchase products. At adult-use dispensaries, the customer needs only to be twenty-one with a state-issued ID in order to purchase cannabis products. Some dispensaries have both a medical side and a recreational side, and each side may offer different products.

DECARBOXYLATION: WHY WE HEAT CANNABIS

In order for the CBD and THC to be activated in cannabis, it needs to be heated. This heating process is called decarboxylation, often shortened to "decarbing." Raw cannabis flowers that come straight from the plant haven't been decarboxylated yet, which means they don't contain CBD or THC (at least, not in large amounts). Raw cannabis contains the precursors to CBD and THC—CBDA and THCA (or "acid cannabinoids"). Raw, non-decarboxylated cannabis will not produce any intoxicating effects, so you probably won't get high if you eat a raw bud (although dried cannabis flowers can naturally decarboxylate over time). When we decarboxylate our cannabis, the CBDA and THCA are converted to CBD and THC. This is the reason people smoke, vape, cook, or otherwise heat cannabis before consuming it. The CBD oils or other cannabis products you purchase at a dispensary or at a store (aside from raw flower) have already been decarboxylated before they reach the shelves. While decarbing is essential for taking advantage of CBD and THC, as we've learned, the CBDA and THCA in the raw cannabis do provide healing benefits as well—they have been shown to have antinausea and anti-inflammatory properties.

METHODS OF DELIVERY FOR CANNABIS MEDICINE

Inhalation

ONSET: IMMEDIATE

DURATION OF EFFECTS: 2–4 HOURS

Inhalation is one of the most common and popular ways to administer cannabis medicine, and the effects are typically felt immediately, or within a few minutes. Due to the quick onset time, inhalation can be very effective for acute situations such as relieving nausea, quick pain relief, stimulating appetite, or reducing anxiety. Inhalation is the fastest delivery method, as the medicine passes through your lungs and into the bloodstream right away. The effects generally last about 2–4 hours, give or take, depending on the person. While inhalation is the quickest-acting, it's also the quickest to fade. So if you're looking for prolonged relief for something like chronic pain or sleep (longer than a couple of hours), a tincture or capsule may be a better bet.

Smoking

Smoking is the most widely known delivery method for consuming cannabis, and you've likely seen it in the form of joints, blunts, pipes, or bowls. Because smoking causes the combustion of the plant material, you may be inhaling chemicals from smoke, tar, and even the butane fumes from your lighter. Therefore, smoking cannabis is not the most highly recommended way to consume it by most cannabis doctors—even if it is the most popular. Smoking can also destroy some of the medicinal cannabinoids and terpenes, which are damaged at higher temperatures. If inhalation is your preferred way to consume cannabis, cannabis doctors often recommend using dry herb vaporizers, which we'll touch on next.

Vaping

Vaporizing (or vaping) is an inhalation method that heats the plant material or an oil to vapor, instead of burning it. It's often considered a healthier way to inhale, as you're avoiding the chemicals in smoke (and preserving more of the terpenes and cannabinoids that could be destroyed in the burning process). While vaping can be discreet and easy, especially with small vape pens, a word of caution—there are a lot of low-quality vape products on the market, and recently reports of vaping-related deaths, illness, and respiratory issues from vaping with tainted oil cartridges have been escalating.

I visited a few licensed dispensaries to ask about the vaping concerns, and while there's still no definite conclusion, the consensus was that the issues with vaping oils come from poor-quality, black-market vape products. Some of these oil vaporizers contain propylene glycol and other chemicals, thinning agents, and synthetic flavor additives that have not been shown to be safe for inhalation. Recently, the Centers for Disease Control and Prevention (CDC) identified vitamin E acetate as a potential ingredient in vape pens causing harm to the lungs in patients diagnosed with vaping illness.

Because investigations are still being done on exactly what is causing the illness and deaths from vaping oils at this time, I would caution against vaping oils in general. If you do decide to vape with oils, make sure to get your vape cartridges from a licensed dispensary and that lab tests have been done on them—so you can be absolutely sure what you're getting.

You can still take advantage of the quick onset of vaporizing by using the dry herb (the raw cannabis flower or "buds") instead of an oil cartridge. I have a dry herb vaporizer at home (mine is the Pax 3), and although it may not be as tiny as vape oil pens, it's a great alternative, as it only has one ingredient—cannabis! You simply pack a small amount of the cannabis flower (as if you were packing a bowl or a joint) right into the vaporizer, and the device heats it up to temperatures that cause vaporization but not combustion. There are many great dry herb vaporizers on the market—including some with a variety of temperature controls—and I expect many more to come as people become more concerned about vaping with oil cartridges.

Sublingual Tinctures

ONSET: ABOUT 15 MINUTES

DURATION OF EFFECTS: 4–6 HOURS

CBD oil is most commonly delivered in tincture form. While the word "tincture" historically refers to an alcohol solution, most CBD and cannabis tinctures today are oil-based and you take them sublingually (under the tongue). The pros of using a tincture include a relatively fast onset time, the second-quickest after inhalation—typically about 15 minutes. With tinctures, it's very easy to measure out a calculated dose, as the oil under your tongue is absorbed into the bloodstream without having to pass through the digestive tract first (as it would with capsules or edibles). Tinctures are easy to carry around with you, a discreet way to administer your cannabis medicine, and the effects typically last longer than inhalation. When you take a tincture, hold it under your tongue (or swish it around in your mouth and let it absorb) for at least 60 seconds before swallowing. If you add your CBD tincture into food or drink, it's delivered into your system as an edible would be, rather than sublingually.

Edibles

ONSET: 60–90 MINUTES

DURATION OF EFFECTS: 6–8 HOURS

"Edibles" refers to anything you eat or drink that contains cannabis (such as pot brownies, or coffee or tea with CBD oil added to it). Edibles and drinkables typically take the longest to produce noticeable effects, but they potentially last the longest, too. Dosing with edibles can be tricky, because they do have to pass through your digestive system before taking effect, and it's hard to know how much medicine your body is absorbing. The effects of edibles can last about 6–8 hours. When you eat a cannabis edible, whether it's CBD, THC, or both, make sure to wait at least an hour, ideally 90 minutes, to feel the effects before deciding if you need more.

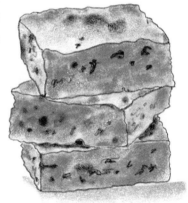

Note: If you're taking your cannabis or CBD medicine by the edible route, avoid gummies with sugar and artificial flavors, as this can negate the anti-inflammatory and antianxiety effects you might be looking for. (If you're a gummy lover, you're in luck: I've shared an awesome, healthy gummy recipe sweetened with honey on page 201).

WHY EDIBLES DELIVER A STRONGER THC EFFECT

If you've ever eaten a cannabis edible, well—you *know*. The effects of an edible with THC in it can feel so much stronger than smoking, using a tincture, or any other method of consuming cannabis. I'd always wondered why THC edibles make people feel so much more stoned than smoking—and it turns out there's a reason.

Even the most experienced cannabis users have stories about accidentally consuming too much of a cannabis edible and not being prepared for the effects. This is because of a surprise guest that pops in when you consume THC edibles—a compound called 11-hydroxy-THC.

11-hydroxy-THC (11-OH-THC) is a metabolite that THC converts to when it passes through the digestive system and the liver (which happens when you eat an edible). It is thought that 11-hydroxy-THC produces much stronger psychoactive effects than those produced by THC alone (although research is inconclusive as to whether the extra-strong high comes directly from 11-OH-THC or the combo of 11-OH-THC and THC together). When THC enters the digestive tract, it passes through the liver before entering the bloodstream. This is known as "first pass effect," which causes even more THC to be converted to 11-hydroxy-THC. Typically, the first pass effect reduces the amount of a drug that makes it into the bloodstream, which lowers the potency—but in the case of THC, it makes the effects stronger. This detour through the digestive system and liver is also the explanation for why it takes longer to feel the effects of THC (and CBD) when you ingest them in food or drink, vs. other delivery methods.

Be aware that if you're planning to consume any type of cannabis with THC in an edible form (this includes capsules or putting drops of a tincture into your food or drink), the THC will be converted to its more psychoactive counterpart. With CBD-only products, this typically isn't a concern, but the more THC in your product, the more 11-hydroxy-THC you'll potentially get once it's digested.

When making the CBD-infused recipes in this book using cannabis that contains higher levels of THC, be extra careful with your dose. As a general rule, stop at just one serving of a THC-rich edible—and make sure to have some non-infused food on hand in case the munchies strike!

Capsules

ONSET: 60-90 MINUTES

DURATION OF EFFECTS: 6-8 HOURS

Capsules are in the same boat as edibles—they take a little bit longer to kick in than inhalation or tinctures. But just like edibles, they tend to last longer than the other delivery methods. I find capsules to be great for sleep, as they last a couple of extra hours longer than the tincture. Like edibles, it can be difficult to dose when using capsules since the CBD has to pass through the digestive tract first—this means that the amount of cannabis medicine that's actually absorbed in the body varies. If you typically experience digestive issues, a tincture may be

a better choice for you, as absorption and
bioavailability will be more streamlined.
On the plus side, capsules are easy to add
to your daily routine if you already take
other pills or supplements, and regardless of
the exact level of absorption, you're still getting
extra cannabinoids into your body and nourishing
your endocannabinoid system.

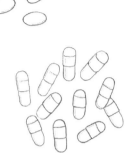

Topicals

ONSET: 10-20 MINUTES

DURATION OF EFFECTS: 2-4 HOURS

Topicals (creams, lotions, oils, salves, or balms) administered directly
on the skin can be fantastic for local pain relief, inflammation, and skin
issues such as rashes, acne, eczema, and psoriasis. Because our skin is
covered with cannabinoid receptors (both CB1 and CB2), many people
find great relief from joint pain and muscle pain from using cannabis
topicals. Topicals typically don't cause any intoxicating effects, even if
they contain high amounts of THC, so this is a perfect way to experience the healing benefits of THC without the high.

Transdermals

ONSET: 10-20 MINUTES

DURATION OF EFFECTS: 2-4 HOURS

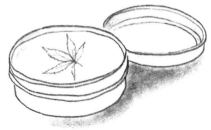

Transdermal products are similar
to topicals—they typically come
as a balm that you rub into your skin,

or as a patch that you apply to the skin—but the medicine can enter the bloodstream rather than providing local relief only (as a topical would). Transdermal compounds or patches may provide deeper pain relief than a topical. With transdermal products there is a bit more of a chance that you'll feel some of the intoxicating effects of THC, since it may enter the bloodstream, but this is usually very slight. One of my favorite products for pain is a transdermal compound with a 1:1 ratio of THC to CBD, which I bought at a dispensary. If you're using a transdermal patch, the recommendation is to place it on a veiny area of the skin, such as the wrist or the inside of the elbow.

Suppositories

ONSET: 10–30 MINUTES

DURATION OF EFFECTS: 4–6 HOURS

Vaginal or rectal suppositories are quickly becoming a popular option for administering CBD, THC, and other cannabinoids as close to the area of need as possible. Suppositories are generally made with CBD (or THC) oil and cocoa butter, and can be used to administer a higher amount of cannabinoids (for menstrual pain, or for cancer patients wanting to take a larger dose of cannabis medicine without feeling the high). The cannabinoids are absorbed directly into the surrounding tissues and can provide pain relief—rarely with any psychoactive effects.

Nano-emulsion/water-soluble CBD: CBD is inherently fat soluble, but companies are beginning to make water-soluble CBD using a process called nano-emulsion. "Nano" means "very small," and nano-emulsion is a process that makes CBD oil molecules tiny enough to be suspended in water. Nano-particles of CBD are reported to have a more efficient level of absorption by the body than regular CBD oil molecules, which makes sense—but don't trust every marketing claim you read when it comes to CBD beverages. The cannabis education site Leafly recently performed a product test on four popular CBD waters, and three out of the four contained no detectable CBD whatsoever. Another great reason to check those lab tests!

HOW LONG CANNABIS STAYS IN THE BODY

The amount of time cannabis remains detectable in the body depends on several factors:

- **Frequency of use**
- **Method of delivery**
- **Personal metabolism**

In non-frequent cannabis users, THC may be undetectable in the body as quickly as twelve days after use. For heavy users, it can stay in your body for as long as thirty days. CBD, on the other hand, has been shown to stay detectable in the body for an average of thirty-seven days.

If you are getting a drug test (which will detect THC metabolites), it's important to remember that full- and broad-spectrum CBD oils may contain trace amounts of THC—so there's always a chance that you will test positive for THC even if you're taking a CBD-only product. You're much less likely to test positive on a drug test from using a CBD isolate, but it's not impossible (as we learned, products are often mislabeled), so you may be better off avoiding cannabis and CBD if THC showing up on a drug test will be a problem for you.

BUT WILL I GET HIGH? USING CANNABIS WITHOUT FEAR

Using Cannabis If You're Sober

I hear from a lot of people in twelve-step addiction-recovery programs who are interested in the benefits of using cannabis therapeutically but don't want to break or threaten their sobriety. I am sensitive to this concern, as I spent the second half of my twenties in twelve-step recovery rooms. I understand the mental, emotional, and physical components of making these choices, which can be extremely challenging to navigate. It's very personal, there is no "right" answer, and the solution will vary from person to person. Many people in sober recovery will be a hard "no" for anything with THC in it, or cannabis in general, as it could be potentially mood-altering. If you are in a sober recovery program, you'll want to take steps to make sure you are 100 percent comfortable with your decision about using cannabis medicine.

Before trying a cannabis product, get very clear about how you feel regarding cannabis in general. Have you had an issue with cannabis use in the past? Do you personally feel that using any part of the cannabis plant, even if it isn't the intoxicating part of the plant, is going to threaten your sobriety or be a "gateway" to participating in other behavior that feels risky to you? Will the smell or taste of cannabis be a negative trigger for you? A good-quality full-spectrum, whole-plant CBD oil might smell and taste like weed and contain trace amounts of THC, so get clear about how this may or may not affect you, mentally and emotionally.

Get really honest about this, journal about it, and make sure to talk about it with a therapist, sponsor, recovery counselor, or someone you trust. Work with that person to create a plan that feels safe and manageable for you.

If you've decided you definitely want to try CBD oil in sobriety but want to avoid THC completely, a broad-spectrum or isolate product may be a good choice for you.

If you do decide to use full-spectrum CBD oil, I suggest starting with a very low dose and paying close attention to how you feel. If you decide to increase your dose, do it very slowly. Once you feel the relief you're looking for, stay at that dose.

If you try a cannabis product, and anything about it doesn't feel right to you or feels threatening to your sobriety, stop using it and get the support you need.

Using Cannabis If You Just Don't Want to Get High

If you're not in a recovery program and you're not worried about threatening your hard-earned sobriety, but you prefer not to feel any psychoactive effects, you have a little bit more room to experiment with your products and dosages. This is the category I fall into today, and I've experimented with my products and dosages enough to understand what amounts and methods of delivery of THC make me feel uncomfortable—if I ever do hit that spot where I *do* feel uncomfortable from the THC, I scale back, and I won't go there again. I have had to experience a few bouts of "Oh, that's a little too much THC" in order to find what works for me. If you want to avoid feeling high, you'll want to focus mainly on CBD-rich products, and nothing with high THC. (Topicals and suppositories are an exception, as they are the least likely to cause intoxicating effects, even at high doses.)

As doctors and experts always say when it comes to cannabis dosing,

"START LOW, AND GO SLOW."

The key to using cannabis without intoxication is to experiment slowly until you find your own personal sweet spot.

If you're using a CBD product, take a small amount to start (5 mg is a good starting point for many people, but for some it's even less) and see how you feel. If you feel fine, no different, or a tiny bit better, and you don't experience anything unpleasant, you can continue to experiment, moving your dose up from there by 5 mg every few days, slowly, if you need to.

If you experience anything unpleasant or uncomfortable when it comes to the THC in the CBD product (such as mental fogginess, anxiety, drowsiness, etc.), you'll know you've hit your upper limit and you can scale back for your next dose (or try a product with less THC in it). You want to allow the cannabis plant to work with you, as your ally—trust that your body will let you know if a certain dosage, product, or cannabis use in general is not the right fit.

If you're comfortable, you can start to move up to a little bit more THC (with products from a dispensary) and see how you feel. Remember, having a little bit of THC in your CBD product can make the CBD work better, and higher THC products can be more therapeutic for some conditions. Work up slowly and mindfully, until you find relief.

Be mindful with your experimentation and document it—including what product you're using and what time of day you take the product, if you take it with food, what level of relief you experience, and any other effects you feel. When it comes to making a decision about using cannabis therapeutics, use your best judgment, pay attention, and rest easy knowing that cannabis is a gentle plant with a high safety profile.

Using Cannabis if You're Not At All Concerned About Getting High

"One person's side effect is another person's benefit," said Michelle Shuffett, MD, National Scientific Director of Columbia Care dispensaries, at the 2019 CannMed conference. This couldn't be more true in the case of cannabis. While some people want to avoid the high completely, others love the feeling of euphoria, relaxation, introspection, sensuality, and even spiritual connection they experience from THC. If you're someone who isn't concerned about the high at all, or you enjoy it, and you want to get the most medicinal and therapeutic benefits possible from your cannabis use, then you have the full freedom to experiment with all kinds of CBD-to-THC ratios until you find the one that gives you the relief you're looking for. Even in this case, it's still important to start low and gradually increase your dose so you can have a clear picture of exactly what works for you, and not overdo it. Cannabis is not a "more is better" type of medicine, so when you feel relief, stay at that dose and enjoy it.

Microdosing THC

When you hear the word "microdosing," psilocybin mushrooms and LSD might be what first come to mind. But there's a whole subset of people out there who microdose THC for its subtle effects on mood and focus. Microdosing with THC is exactly what it sounds like— taking very tiny amounts of THC that don't make you feel high but slightly alter and enhance your experience.

However, as Dr. Bonni Goldstein says, "A microdose of THC is actually just a *dose*," as some people need only the tiniest doses of THC to find the relief they're looking for.

When I started experimenting with tiny amounts of THC, I used a tincture that was very specifically dosed to be 1 mg per drop of oil. I used only one drop under my tongue, and the effects were really nice— even for someone like me who avoids the THC high. I was able to focus more efficiently, and I felt more creative while I was writing. I noticed that the taste of food was just slightly enhanced, and the music I was listening to was slightly more enjoyable—yet I wasn't impaired or stoned at all.

Microdosing THC can also be a great way to get acquainted with how THC makes you feel if you're unsure about it or haven't had THC in a long time. Taking 1 mg of THC may make you feel absolutely nothing different, but if you're anything like me, it just might *slightly* enhance your day. Everyone is different with how they react to THC, so you may enjoy the effects of a few more milligrams—or you may want to just stick with CBD only. This is where the magic happens— when you can use cannabis strategically to enhance your life without feeling any uncomfortable effects. You can create whatever experience you want to have with it. Please know that I'm not recommending experimenting with THC if you're sober, or otherwise THC-averse.

If you do want to try microdosing THC, I recommend using a tincture, which makes it super easy to manage your dose. You can literally create your experience drop by drop. Start with one drop and go about your day. Make sure to wait at least thirty minutes to let the effects kick in before taking another drop—I usually recommend waiting fifteen minutes with CBD, but with THC you really don't want to overdo it. I wouldn't recommend microdosing with edibles, because they take so long to kick in, and the absorption and effects can be more unpredictable.

Consumed Too Much THC? Here's What to Do

THC is known to cause euphoria and can be mood-enhancing, pain-relieving, and relaxing at the right levels—but it can also cause anxiety and paranoia if too much is consumed.

CBD, if it's present in the cannabis strain in high enough amounts, can safeguard you from these unwanted effects of THC, so choosing a higher-CBD product can mitigate the high.

Cannabis strains that are high in the terpenes limonene, pinene, and caryophyllene can also bring down the mental fogginess from THC—which explains why lemon, black pepper, and pine (including eating pine nuts!) can be helpful in reducing the high.

If you get too high, Dr. Ethan Russo has recommended having terpene-rich foods on hand that can help bring down THC's effects. I love this idea, because it's something delicious you can lean on (or make for your friends) during too-much-THC times of need. He recommends eating pesto (with lots of pine nuts, for the pinene) and drinking lemonade with extra lemon zest from the rinds (which contain limonene). Dr. Russo recommends having these foods prepared and on hand in your fridge *before* you consume any cannabis, because once you've had too much THC you may have difficulty preparing them. At the very least, even if you don't have these recipes prepared, make sure to have some lemons, black pepper, and pine nuts on hand if you're having a gathering where cannabis products are being consumed. This could be a really fun party favor—a jar of homemade pesto or a bottle of homemade lemonade. What's better than that, even if you *aren't* getting high?

Tips if you've consumed too much THC:

- Sleep it off (take a nap if you can).
- Drink water.
- Take a shower.
- Chew on black peppercorns (which contain caryophyllene).

- Drink lemonade with extra lemon zest (which contains limonene) or smell lemon essential oil.

- Eat pine nuts (which contain pinene; see recipe for pesto that follows).

- Take CBD to mitigate THC's effects (although CBD may more effectively inhibit the high when taken *before* THC).

- Take a walk in nature (make sure you're in a place where you feel safe, or with a friend).

- Watch a favorite movie, write in a journal, or listen to a favorite album.

- Breathe, relax, and know the effects will lift soon.

CBD PESTO

This terpene-rich pesto is great for any occasion. You're getting limonene from the lemon, pinene from the pine nuts, and caryophyllene from the black pepper. You'll learn how to make CBD-infused olive oil on page 140, which you can use in this recipe—or keep it simple and use a few dropperfuls of your favorite unflavored CBD oil tincture. To make this recipe dairy-free, skip the parmesan.

Makes 2 cups of pesto

2 cloves garlic

1 cup fresh basil

½ cup pine nuts

Juice of 1 lemon

1 tsp. lemon zest

¼ cup freshly grated Parmesan

Salt and freshly ground black pepper to taste

½ cup CBD-infused olive oil, recipe on page 140 (or ½ cup plain olive oil + a few dropperfuls of your CBD oil tincture, unflavored)

Add all ingredients except the olive oil to your blender or food processor. Pulse all ingredients together and add olive oil slowly, until the pesto reaches your desired consistency. When pesto is mixed to your liking, use it as a sauce or dip, or drizzle over your favorite savory dish.

CBD LEMONADE

This homemade lemonade will harness the uplifting powers of limonene to brighten your mood and your day. For a lower sugar version, try it with a few drops of liquid stevia instead of honey.

Makes 2 cups of lemonade

Juice of 2 lemons

1 tsp. lemon zest

2 cups water

1 tsp. raw honey

1 dropperful of your favorite CBD oil

Put all ingredients in blender, blend, and serve over ice.

CANNABIS AND CBD DOSING: A PRIMER

Dosing! This is the part you've been waiting for, right? Most people ask the same question when it comes to CBD or cannabis therapeutics in general: "How much should I take for my specific condition?" When researching for this book, I was determined to get a definite answer for this—I searched tirelessly to find the holy grail of dosing recommendations. As it turns out, it's not that simple—the right dose requires personalization and finesse.

Each cannabis expert I talked to or researched said the same thing—it's more about treating the *person* than the specific condition. Using cannabis medicine effectively requires that you get intimately acquainted with how you feel, so you can adjust your dose as you need to based on your unique sensitivity and needs.

The right cannabis and CBD dosing protocol is influenced by a variety of factors, including:

- Your individual sensitivity to cannabis, particularly CBD and THC
- Your cannabis experience and tolerance
- The type of cannabis product you're consuming (full-spectrum, broad-spectrum, isolate)
- The quality of the product
- The ratio of CBD to THC in the product
- The method of delivery (tincture, topical, edible, capsule, inhalation)
- The time of day you use it

- What kind of relief (and the degree of relief) you're looking for

MY VISIT WITH A CANNABIS DOCTOR

To learn more about dosing and to understand how a cannabis doctor works with patients, I took a trip to Maine to visit Dr. Dustin Sulak at his practice, Integr8 Health. He's advised thousands of patients on how to use cannabis therapeutically, and is dedicated to educating patients, caregivers, and clinicians about cannabis medicine online at Healer.com. I've found Dr. Sulak's work to be extremely helpful in learning to use cannabis for myself, and helping to manage my dad's cannabis regimen—so I was excited to visit his office and learn from him directly.

HOW DOES A CANNABIS MEDICINE PRACTICE WORK?

When Dr. Sulak's patients come in to see him at his office, they tell him what they're struggling with and he gives them detailed recommendations on how cannabis might best support their needs. First, he informs each patient about the risks and benefits, then helps them to get started on a treatment plan. It isn't unlike Dr. Frank Lipman's functional medicine practice in New York City, where I used to work as a health coach—except we didn't work with cannabis.

Dr. Sulak says the number one condition he sees patients for is chronic pain—but he also sees patients with PTSD, cancer, neurologic disorders, inflammatory conditions, Crohn's disease, rheumatoid arthritis, pediatric seizures, and pediatric cancers.

"We're a magnet for conditions that fail to respond to conventional medicine, and we have incredible results. Most of our new patients now are either older adults or very young children," he says.

He feels strongly about treating the individual human, not only their symptoms, which is a major tenet of functional and integrative medicine. This means that he takes everything about their current lifestyle into consideration.

When meeting with a new patient he'll ask these questions before making specific cannabis recommendations:

- If you could get anything out of this visit, what would it be?
- If you were much healthier in two months, how would life be different? Please paint the picture for me.
- How well are you sleeping?
- Please describe your diet. What did you eat yesterday?

All of these answers have a place in an integrative practice, and cannabis medicine can play a role in helping patients to feel well and balanced again.

Once Dr. Sulak and his patient come up with a plan about how cannabis may work best for them, the patient gets certified to receive their medical cannabis card. At that point, the patient or their chosen caregiver can go to a medical cannabis dispensary to purchase cannabis medicine.

Dr. Sulak recommends patients start with a very low dose of cannabis and work their way up until they find their personal "therapeutic window"—the sweet spot that gives them the perfect amount of relief, but without any uncomfortable effects.

While THC is "more potent and powerful," CBD is "more forgiving," explains Dr. Sulak, which means you can experiment with a higher dose of CBD than you can with THC, without experiencing discomfort. Adding CBD to the THC "makes THC's therapeutic window wider," so many of his patients can tolerate a higher dose of THC if CBD is there with it.

Using CBD alone can get expensive if you're taking high doses— but "if you sprinkle a little bit of THC in there, you can get a more powerful dose that works beautifully, without bumping up the price," says Dr. Sulak. "Mother Nature gives them to us together for a reason."

He calls CBD a "promiscuous substance," meaning it does many different things in the body—it can be anti-pain, antispasm, anti-inflammatory, and antianxiety, and it helps the body to regulate itself and stay in balance. Dr. Sulak says CBD is "extraordinarily safe," even at very high doses.

He is particularly enthusiastic about the acid cannabinoids in the cannabis plant—that is, CBDA and THCA—the non-intoxicating compounds in the plant that are present before the plant is heated. The acid cannabinoids have many of the same anti-inflammatory benefits of CBD and THC, and may be more bioavailable (better absorbed by the body), so there's no need for large or expensive doses.

In order to take advantage of these acid cannabinoids that are present in raw, unheated cannabis, Dr. Sulak recommends making a raw cannabis tea. In fact, he makes this tea for himself most mornings.

To make raw cannabis tea, you take a small bud of fresh, dried cannabis flower (you only need a tiny bit, the size of a pea) and pour hot water over it.

Steep it for 5 minutes, then drink it as you would any tea. You can add this pea-sized bud of cannabis to any hot beverage. The heat from the hot water will not cause enough decarboxylation, typically, to cause the acid cannabinoids to turn into THC or CBD—so there's very little chance of feeling psychoactive effects. After you drink your cannabis tea, "you can just chew up that little bud at the bottom of your mug and eat it," Dr. Sulak says.

For the cannabis tea, he recommends using Type 2 cannabis, which has close to an equal ratio of CBD to THC, so you can get the benefits of both CBDA and THCA in your tea.

CANNABIS MEDICINE: FINDING YOUR DOSE

When considering cannabis medicine and trying to find your own therapeutic window, it can be helpful to find a local cannabis doctor to work with. A cannabis doctor can help you safely find an appropriate starting dose and help you make a plan for how often you should (if necessary) titrate your dose up.

When finding your personal therapeutic window, the difference may be just a few milligrams. Resist the urge to believe that more is always better. You'll likely want to start way lower than you think you should, especially if you're sensitive.

"The goal is to use the minimal amount of cannabis to achieve the maximum benefits. You know you've reached your optimal dose when you feel enough symptom relief that you are no longer limited by whatever was bothering you," says Dr. Sulak.

Although 1 mg (or even less) can be the optimal starting point for THC dosing for some patients, the starting point for CBD tends to be a little bit higher. Dr. Caroline MacCallum, who has a medical cannabis practice based in Canada, says she usually uses a starting dose of 5–10 mg of CBD with her patients.

Dr. Bonni Goldstein says that in her cannabis practice in Los Angeles, the dose can vary a lot from patient to patient—even in patients with the same condition. While one patient may do really well on a dose of 4 mg of CBD, another may need 400 mg to find relief. In regard to finding your perfect dose, Dr. Goldstein says, "If you see no change, you haven't found your dose yet. If you experience a negative side effect, your dose may be too high, or you're not using the right chemovar (strain) or product."

There is often a bell curve, or "biphasic effect," with cannabis medicine, meaning that some of the effects that can be helpful at low doses can make things feel worse at higher doses. A tiny bit of THC may be helpful for sleep or anxiety, but at higher doses it may heighten anxiety or disrupt sleep. Same goes for CBD—a larger amount of CBD can sometimes be *less* effective than a small or moderate dose.

Frequent check-ins about how you're feeling, along with tracking the different products you try in a journal, can be crucial to finding what cannabis product and dose works best for your condition and expectations.

"Ten milligrams of CBD may be a great dose for general wellness," Dr. Sulak said. "That amount can be incredible for mood-boosting, relieving pain and anxiety, and balancing out the system. People who are in severe pain may need a higher dose, perhaps fifty and two hundred milligrams, to feel relief. The same goes for severe anxiety."

Of course, this will differ from person to person and from product to product, so personal experimentation is king.

To find the right dose for you, it's important to notice how you feel *before* taking your cannabis medicine. Dr. Sulak has a practice he calls the Inner Inventory.

How to Check Your Inner Inventory (© Dustin Sulak):

RATE EACH ON A SCALE OF 1 TO 10 (1 = WORST AND 10 = BEST) BEFORE AND
1-2 HOURS AFTER TAKING EACH DOSE. SET AN ALARM REMINDER AND
RECORD YOUR SCORES FOR BEST RESULTS.

- BREATH: How easy and smooth is your breath?

- BODY: How comfortable and calm does your body feel?
  How easy is it to remain still and comfortable?

- MOOD: How easy is it for you to feel a sense of
  contentment and appreciation? How easy is it for you to
  smile right now?

- SYMPTOMS: How severe are your symptoms? (1 = minimal
  and 10 = severe)

Dr. Sulak's recommendations on finding your therapeutic window
for any cannabis product are as follows:

- **Inhalation.** Take one inhalation and wait 5–10 minutes before
  deciding if you need more.

- **Tincture.** Take the lowest dose (as low as 1–2 mg for THC, or
  5 mg for CBD) and wait 30–60 minutes before deciding if
  you need more.

- **Edibles** (this includes capsules). Take the lowest dose and
  wait 2–4 hours before deciding if you need more.

After consuming the cannabis, take note if your inner inventory
score has improved. If so, this means you're on the right track to finding your optimal dose. Be patient, pay attention to your body and
mind, and only increase your dose if you don't feel any relief.

CBD-TO-THC RATIOS

One of the best ways to find your therapeutic window if you have access to a wide range of CBD products is to experiment with the amount of THC that you can comfortably tolerate. You may find you feel better with a high-CBD, low-THC product, or you may find that a balanced 1:1 ratio of CBD to THC works better for you, depending on your condition.

When I met Martin A. Lee from Project CBD, he told me that in California, the dispensaries have a vast array of products with different CBD-to-THC ratios—*way* more choices than in a state that has access to only hemp-derived CBD.

There's one cannabis product producer in particular called Canna-Craft, in the San Francisco Bay Area, that he thought I should check out if I wanted to know more about product ratios and see how CBD oil is made. Continuing my quest to find the holy grail of dosing, I headed out to San Francisco to meet with Martin and take a tour of CannaCraft.

When I landed in San Francisco, I first went to three different dispensaries and got a variety of products to experiment with. At the time of this writing, California has adult-use legal dispensaries where you can purchase a number of cannabis products at different CBD-to-THC ratios, without having to go through the process of getting a medical card. Going into a cannabis dispensary in California made me feel like a kid in a candy store—and I don't even like to get high! I also learned that proper dosing is often less about the actual milligrams you're taking, and more about the CBD-to-THC ratio that works best for you. Your own sensitivity to THC will ultimately be the deciding factor in which product and ratio are optimal.

"This is one of the many gifts of CBD: It can magnify the medicinal impact of a small amount of THC so that one need not consume an intoxicating dose to experience THC's therapeutic benefits," says Lee, who has been instrumental in helping to develop some of the most commonly used CBD-to-THC ratios in cannabis therapeutics in California. I got a much better sense of how this works when we went over to the CannaCraft to take a tour. They manufacture Care By Design CBD products, with a wide array of different CBD-to-THC ratios to choose from, so people have access to personalized medicine.

If you have access to a range of cannabis tinctures and capsules with various CBD-to-THC ratios where you live, here are some guidelines on ratios:

WHEN YOU SEE A CBD-TO-THC RATIO LIKE 30:1, THAT MEANS THERE'S 30 MG OF CBD FOR EVERY 1 MG OF THC IN THE PRODUCT. THE FOLLOWING ARE COMMON RATIOS AVAILABLE AT LICENSED DISPENSARIES IN CALIFORNIA. YOU MAY SEE DIFFERENT RATIOS AT YOUR DISPENSARY, BUT THESE GENERAL GUIDELINES WILL STILL HOLD TRUE.

30:1, 20:1, or 18:1. These ratios are for those looking for the healing effects of CBD, without the high of THC. At higher ratios of CBD, balance can be provided to the endocannabinoid system without any intoxicating effects. Many people use these ratios for mood, anxiety, pain, inflammation, and general daytime use. The small amounts of THC in these products can boost the healing properties of the CBD.

10:1. Although everyone will have a different experience, a ratio of

10:1 CBD to THC or higher is what most experts generally recommend as the baseline for someone who doesn't want to feel the intoxicating effects of THC. New cannabis users or sensitive people may experience a bit of a high from this ratio, so it's recommended to use it at night, or on a low-pressure day, especially if you're trying it for the first time.

8:1 and 4:1. These ratios are best suited to people who have some experience with THC, or whose symptoms respond better to more THC. Some people find these ratios helpful for pain and sleep. Novice or sensitive cannabis users may feel some psychoactive effects from the THC at these ratios.

2:1 and 1:1. These are more balanced ratios of CBD to THC, and can be psychoactive even at smaller doses. Many people find these ratios helpful for treating pain, inflammation, and sleep problems, as they can have a more sedative effect. Some consider a 1:1 ratio to be the most "medicinal" of all the ratios, since the CBD and THC are represented in equal amounts. If you have a serious condition and want to get more cannabinoids into your system, you can titrate your dose up slowly without increasing your high. Continue to titrate up slowly, drop by drop, or milligram by milligram. (*Sources: Care By Design and Proof Extracts.*)

CBD Only (no THC). Some people report success for anxiety, pain, and epilepsy with CBD that contains zero THC, but they may require higher doses to have an effect, because of the lack of THC and other cannabinoids and terpenes.

THC Only (no CBD). Typically for users who enjoy the intoxicating, euphoric effects of THC—can be effective for pain and nausea, and can be useful in topicals without intoxicating effects.

Everyone will respond differently to different ratios of CBD to
THC, but if I could magically place a bottle of cannabis oil in
everyone's home for general wellness, I'd pick a 1:1 ratio.

—*Dr. Dustin Sulak*

Guidelines for Finding Your Optimal Dose

- **Pick a CBD-to-THC ratio to start with.** If you're sensitive or
  new to using cannabis, start with a higher CBD-to-THC ratio—
  typically, a full-spectrum hemp-derived CBD oil, or a CBD oil
  with ratios of 10:1 or higher (10:1, 18:1, 20:1 and up) is not likely
  to produce intoxicating effects.

- **Start with the lowest dose.** Often, the recommended starting
  point is between 2.5 and 5 mg of CBD, and 1–2 mg of THC.
  Keep in mind that for sensitive people, just 2 mg of THC can be
  the "psychoactive threshold," so if you don't want to feel high,
  start lower. Remember, a higher amount of CBD will lessen the
  intoxicating effects of THC.

- **Keep your dose the same for a few days before adding more
  or changing the ratio.** After two to three days, if you're using a
  product with THC in it, increase your dose by about 1–2 mg (per
  Dr. Ethan Russo), and continue with slow dose escalation until
  you find optimal relief. With high-CBD products that contain
  little to no THC, you can typically be more generous with dose
  increase, increasing by 5 mg at a time.

- **Pay close attention to how you feel.** Keep a journal to note how
  you feel before and after, the time of day, and what dose and ratio
  you took.

- **Experiment with different methods of delivery.** You may prefer
  the soothing pain relief of a topical, the immediate relief of

inhalation, the fast-acting and calming effects of a tincture, or the slow, longer-lasting effects of a capsule or edible.

- **If you experience any negative effects from THC**, consider switching to a higher-CBD product, lowering your THC dose, or choosing a different method of delivery that suits you better.

CBD DOSING QUICK GUIDE

Some general guidelines for CBD products (with little to no THC):

- A small dose is typically between 1 and 15mg
- A standard dose is typically between: 15 and 75 mg
- A large dose is typically 75 mg+

Start with 2.5–5 mg (a very small/conservative dose for most people) and work your way up as needed until you feel relief. When you do feel relief, stay at that dose.

HOW TO GET STARTED WITH CBD IF . . .

You're in a non-legal state or you have access only to hemp-derived CBD:

- **Get a lab test.** Because CBD is currently highly unregulated (as of 2020), there are a lot of products out there that don't contain the amount of CBD they say they contain, claim to be full-spectrum or whole-plant but are actually just isolate, or are otherwise making false marketing claims. If you request a third-party lab test, you should check to make sure the amount of

CBD is accurate (does the lab test match the label?), that other cannabinoids and terpenes are in the product (if it's advertised as full-spectrum, broad-spectrum, or whole-plant), and that it tested negative for heavy metals, pesticides, and solvents. You'll also want to see how much THC is in your product. Even though .3 percent is the legal limit, some companies have been found to add higher amounts, and some have zero—even if they claim to be full-spectrum. I always like to know what I'm taking, so I almost always ask for a lab test before trying a new CBD oil. To get a lab test, check the company's website or contact the company directly.

- **Try a tincture.** If you get the lab test and trust that your product is high-quality, try a few drops of a tincture under your tongue and see how you feel. Because there is little to no THC in your CBD product, you don't have to necessarily start with the low starting point (1–2 mg) that you would with a THC product. You could start at 5–10 mg and see if you feel any effects. Tinctures are great because you can accurately calculate your dose based on how many milligrams are in 1 ml (a dropperful) of your CBD tincture, and over a few days, find the dose that works for you.

- **Try a capsule.** Not thrilled with the tincture route, and want to see how a capsule might feel? Many companies that make tinctures also have capsules available. It can take an hour or more to feel relief from a capsule, so keep that in mind if you're looking for instant relief.

- **Consider inhalation for the quickest relief.** In my experience, the best way to truly understand how CBD is different from THC is to take an inhalation of CBD flower, preferably with a dry herb vaporizer. Most people report an almost instant feeling of calm, and anxiety melting away, when vaporizing or smoking the dry herb—but with no high. It's very different from what most people experience when smoking or vaping high-THC cannabis.

- **Try a CBD topical.** I love CBD topicals for pain, and although I find they work better for me when there's more THC in there, CBD-only (or very-low-THC) topicals often work great, too—especially for joint pain or arthritis. Many people swear by CBD topicals for the skin, too, as they can help to soothe and calm inflammation.

- **Make your own edibles.** If you really want to go to the next level, you can buy dried CBD flower (the dried buds that are typically used for smoking) and infuse it into butter, olive oil, or coconut oil—and use it in your cooking. For an overview on how to make these delicious CBD-infused creations, turn to the Cooking with Cannabis section (page 133). I don't recommend buying most pre-made edibles, as they are often loaded with sugar or corn syrup and artificial colors and flavors, which defeats the purpose of trying to lower your inflammation or calm your anxiety.

If You're in a State with Legal Medical Cannabis

If you're in a state where you need a medical card to obtain any products with higher than .3 percent THC, consider getting a medical card. Some states have stricter regulations than others about who is eligible for the medical program. You'll need to visit a cannabis doctor to get started with that process.

How to Get a Medical Card:
The exact procedure will vary state by state, but in general:

- Find a cannabis doctor near you (search online for "cannabis doctor in [insert your city here]").

- Make an appointment with a doctor and get approved for your card (each state will have its own regulations on which conditions qualify for approval). There will be a fee for this appointment, which varies by doctor, and you will likely have to renew your medical card annually.

- You will submit the approval (or the doctor will submit the approval for you) to your state's medical cannabis program, and then you will receive your medical card in the mail (and most likely, a temporary card to use in the meantime).

- You should have the option to assign a caregiver to your account, who can pick up your cannabis medicine for you.

- Take your medical card with you to a licensed dispensary (this is where you will obtain your cannabis products) and talk to the budtenders there about your needs. Your cannabis doctor can recommend the best dispensaries in the area. If your doctor gave you a prescription with specific product recommendations, or any other documentation about your visit, bring that documentation with you to the dispensary in case you need it.

Once you have your medical card and can access a dispensary:

- **First, get clear on what kind of relief you're looking for,** and how you'll know when you feel it. Are you looking to calm your anxiety? Reduce your pain? Help with sleep?

- **Consider starting with a high-CBD tincture or capsule (such as** 20:1 or 18:1 CBD to THC) and begin with the smallest dose to test your sensitivity to the THC.

- **If you're an experienced cannabis user or dealing with a serious condition** and you know you want higher levels of THC, you can experiment with something higher—such as a 1:1 ratio—and see how you feel.

- **Keep a journal.** Write down how you felt before taking the cannabis medicine, what dose you took, how long it took to feel the effects, and how it made you feel.

- **Understand that different methods of delivery are good for different conditions.** You may find a tincture helps you with daily anxiety, a topical helps you with pain, and a capsule or edible helps you with sleep. Or you may find something completely different. Experiment with a few different methods, and pay close attention to how your mind and body feel.

If you're in an "adult-use" (aka "recreational") legal state:

- **If you're in an adult-use legal state,** you're in luck—you likely have access to a full range of CBD products with different THC ratios, without needing to get a medical card (although this isn't always the case—some states have different products at medical dispensaries than they do at recreational dispensaries).

- **If this is the case, look up a few different dispensaries near you**—I recommend checking out more than one, if you have access to options. Dispensaries will often have different product offerings, so you may find one dispensary that has the suppositories or transdermal compounds you want, and another dispensary has high-CBD flower for your dry herb vaporizer or infusing into edibles. Most dispensaries will have their menu available on their website, and many of them change their websites frequently to represent their current product offerings.

- **Try a variety of methods of delivery and CBD-to-THC ratios, as mentioned above.** Have fun with it, knowing that you may have to try different doses and methods of delivery to find your personal sweet spot.

TRIED CBD AND IT DIDN'T WORK? THIS MIGHT BE WHY

If you tried a CBD product and it didn't work for you, or you felt nothing, here are a few reasons why this could be. CBD (and cannabis in general) isn't for everyone, so if it doesn't agree with you or doesn't seem to give you the relief you're looking for, it could be that cannabis isn't for you. It's not a magic bullet for everything. That's okay (and, hey, you can still try mushrooms)!

Everybody's endocannabinoid system is unique, just like everyone's digestive system is unique. It's hard to say that there's one food that's good for everyone's digestion across the board. What makes one person feel soothed could make another feel bloated. In the same way, a certain dosage of CBD may make me sleepy, but it may make you alert. While a certain level of THC may make one person feel calm, it may make another feel anxious. Using cannabis therapeutically is a delicate and intricate process.

If you tried CBD and didn't feel anything, here are a few potential reasons:

- **You took an isolate.** CBD isolates definitely have their place, but for many people, they don't work as effectively as full-spectrum products. If you tried CBD and you didn't feel any relief, consider switching to a full-spectrum CBD product. The compounds in cannabis work more effectively together.

- **You didn't take the correct dose.** With any cannabis medicine, the goal is to find your own personal "therapeutic window." Take note of what dose you took, and experiment with different doses of CBD. You'll likely need to play with the dosing a bit to feel the relief you're looking for.

- **Your product isn't what it says it is.** Get a lab test. Your tincture may say each dropperful has 25 mg of CBD in it, but the lab test could show a different amount. Find a product where the label matches the lab test for more accurate dosing.

- **Your method of delivery wasn't correct for your needs.** Maybe you tried a topical when a tincture or capsule would be better for what you're looking for. Maybe you inhaled using a CBD vaporizer, but you were looking for something longer-lasting. Maybe you tried an edible, and the way it reacted with your digestive system didn't deliver the effects you were hoping for. Try a different method and see what happens!

- **You were taking too many things at once.** For your first few experiences with CBD or cannabis medicine, I would highly recommend you take it alone, or have it be the one thing you do differently—not at the exact same time as other new herbs or supplements. It will be easier for you to feel what's happening in your body if you introduce new things one at a time.

- **The cannabinoid and terpene profile in the product wasn't ideal for your needs.** As you begin to navigate the world of cannabis therapeutics and try products with different cannabinoid and terpene profiles, you'll find the products and strains you prefer. Leafly.com is a fantastic resource for investigating the cannabinoid and terpene profiles in a variety of the most popular cannabis strains—including high-CBD strains.

After all of my personal experimentation over the past couple of years, I've found that my favorite two methods of delivery are tinctures and topicals. This is because tinctures are extremely easy to dose—you can experiment with them *drop by drop* until you find a dose that works well for you. Topicals are fantastic, particularly for pain relief, because there are rarely any intoxicating effects. Edibles and inhalation tend to be more difficult to dose (unless you're using a vaporizer that comes with exact dosing measurements).

WHEN YOU WALK INTO A DISPENSARY FOR THE FIRST TIME

Budtenders (the friendly people behind the counter at the dispensary) are great to talk to about your needs, and there are many highly knowledgeable budtenders out there. I've spent a lot of time hanging out at dispensaries over the past two years, chatting with budtenders, and I love hearing their stories about what works for them and their customers. That being said, a budtender may not be equipped to give recommendations on your specific condition (especially if you're not at a medical dispensary), so you should always walk in with enough of your own research done to make an informed decision.

Here are a few questions to answer before your first dispensary trip:

- What symptoms are you hoping to relieve with cannabis?
- How comfortable are you with feeling the high from THC?
- Do you want something with CBD only, or are you comfortable with trying out different ratios?
- What is your preferred method of delivery?

- Check the dispensary's menu online, if they have one. Are there specific products you know you want to try?

Answering these questions for yourself will help you facilitate conversations with your budtender and make it easier to find the right products for you.

WHO SHOULDN'T USE CANNABIS THERAPEUTICALLY?

There are a few circumstances when it's particularly important to be cautious when using cannabis therapeutically. If you're not sure whether or not cannabis is right for you, my suggestion is to consult a cannabis doctor, especially in the following cases:

- **Pregnancy and breastfeeding.** Although cannabis has been used gynecologically for centuries, there have not been enough studies done to show the safety of using cannabis products during pregnancy and breastfeeding. For this reason, most doctors recommend avoiding it until more research is done. If you're considering cannabis medicine for a child or teenager, work closely with a cannabis doctor who has experience with pediatric patients.

- **Schizophrenia, panic attacks, or other mental health conditions.** While high-CBD products can sometimes be helpful in these cases, high-THC use can cause anxiety paranoia and potentially exacerbate symptoms of schizophrenia in some patients. If you have a history or predisposition to schizophrenia, panic attacks, or any mental health condition, work with cannabis medicine only under a doctor's close supervision.

- **Immunotherapy.** Although cannabis has been shown to be a great help when it comes to chemotherapy and cancer treatment, a study on patients going through immunotherapy treatments showed that cannabis made the immunotherapy drugs less effective (but the cannabis did not have a negative impact on overall disease outcome). If you are going through immunotherapy for cancer and considering using cannabis, work closely with a doctor and monitor your progress with frequent check-ins.

Check the Memorial Sloan Kettering site of mskcc.org to look for potential drug interactions with your current medications before using cannabis.

CBD AND PETS

Many owners of furry friends swear by giving their dogs CBD for anxiety, pain, and hyperactivity. If your pup is in need of some soothing and calming, many companies make CBD tinctures developed especially for dogs. In most cases, these tinctures are the same as the ones made for humans, but typically in smaller doses. You can give your pet a tincture directly into the mouth, or you can add CBD oil to your pet's food or treats. A 2018 study showed significant pain relief in dogs with a dosage of 2 mg/kg twice a day, without side effects, and another in 2019 showed a decrease in seizures in dogs who were given 2.5 mg/kg of CBD twice a day.

Based on these studies, if you have a 20 lb. (9 kg) pet, the dose would be about 18–20 mg of CBD twice a day.

Many experts and CBD companies that make pet products suggest starting at a lower dose, however, and working your way up to the dose that's best for your pet, just as you would with a human dose.

Lazarus Naturals, a Colorado-based CBD company that has a line of pet tinctures, recommends the following starting doses based on weight for pets.

- Less than 15 lbs.: 3 drops (1.5 mg)
- 15–30 lbs.: 6 drops (3 mg)
- 30–60 lbs.: 10 drops (5 mg)
- Over 60 lbs.: 20 drops (10 mg)

Just like you would with a human, start slow and titrate up as needed based on how your pet responds.

For more of my favorite cannabis books, resources, and brands, head to the Resources section.

> Cannabis is the single most versatile herbal remedy, and the most useful plant on Earth. No other single plant contains as wide a range of medically active herbal constituents.
>
> —Dr. Ethan Russo

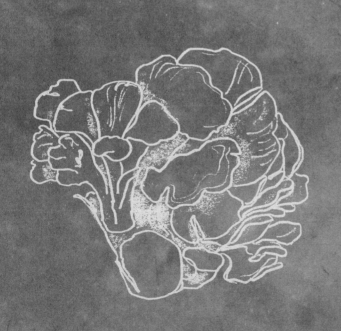

MEET THE MEDICINAL MUSHROOMS

Now that you're officially acquainted with cannabis, it's time to meet the other group of all-stars to add to your Rebel's Apothecary—the mushrooms! I'm tempted to call all of the medicinal mushrooms in this book "magic" mushrooms, because they're all pretty magical, but we'll be covering psychedelic mushrooms later in the book—so I'll save the "magic" distinction for those. However, the medicinal mushrooms you're about to meet have an incredible array of healing powers.

Medicinal mushrooms (also called functional mushrooms) have been used traditionally for thousands of years as powerful healers to promote well-being and longevity. These mushrooms can help strengthen your immune system, lower inflammation, prevent disease, sharpen your mind, give you more energy, calm your nervous system, help you sleep better at night, and potentially even fight cancer.

The world of mycology (which means the study of fungi) is so much more fascinating than I ever could have imagined. Mushrooms have astonishing powers, and I'm excited to share them with you—so you can start to form your own healing relationship with fungi.

MUSHROOMS AREN'T ACTUALLY PLANTS

First things first—did you know that mushrooms aren't actually plants? That's right—they're fungi, and they have their own fungi *kingdom!* You and I reside in the animal kingdom, cannabis lives in the plant kingdom, and mushrooms belong to the fungi kingdom. In fact, researchers have found that mushrooms are more genetically similar to animals than plants.

Not only do mushrooms help us stay healthy as humans, but they play an instrumental role in the health of the planet. Mushrooms have been shown to excrete enzymes that break down the hydrocarbon bonds in plastic, and therefore can help clean toxins from the environment and the soil (a process known as mycoremediation). Trust me— mushrooms are much more interesting than just something you might find at a salad bar.

Let's start with the fungi basics. There are three parts of the mushroom you'll want to get familiar with—the mycelium, the fruiting body, and the spores. First, we'll cover the root system of the mushroom—the mycelium. Mycelium is arguably one of the most important substances on this planet.

MUSHROOM MYCELIUM

Walk through any forest and you'll probably see a mushroom or two growing under a tree or on a log—but the largest part of the fungi kingdom is actually hidden from our sight. Those beautiful mushrooms you see peeking out from the dirt are connected to an intricate network of underground roots called "mycelium." The mycelium of the mushroom kingdom lives underground, weaving its way through-out the root systems of every forest on Earth. These roots span for miles around the globe, and are responsible for not only delivering nutrients to mushrooms and surrounding trees and plants but also for cleaning the soil and decomposing toxins and dead trees throughout the forest.

The mycelium is known as the neurological network of the forest—mushroom expert Paul Stamets, author of *Mycelium Running*, refers to mycelium as the Earth's "natural Internet." This mushroom myce-lium is connected to the root systems of trees and other plants, and they trade nutrients with one another. Mushroom mycelium looks like tiny white threads—you might be able to find some just by going out into the forest and digging your hand into the woodchips under your feet. If you see tiny white strands running through the soil, you've found mycelium.

THE FRUITING BODY

The fruiting body is the part you likely think of when you imagine a mushroom—it's the part that sprouts up from the ground, and it's the "meaty" part of the mushroom we cook and eat. When you buy mush-rooms at the grocery store, what you're buying is the fruiting body. The fruiting body is made of condensed mycelium—it's the reproductive structure of the mycelium. The fruiting body of the mushroom con-tains medicinal compounds called beta-glucans, which are naturally occurring polysaccharides. These are the compounds known for being able to modulate the immune system, and they are responsible for many of the healing properties of the mushrooms.

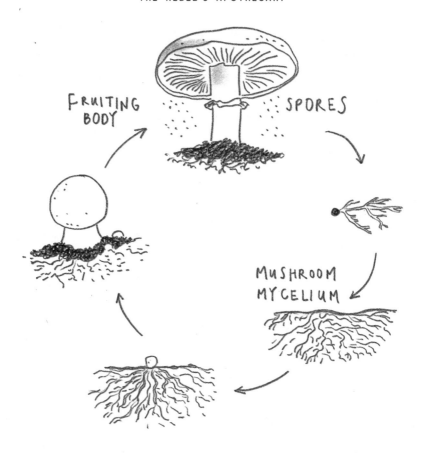

SPORES

We can't talk about the mycelium and the fruiting body without addressing the very way mushrooms replicate themselves—with their spores. Mushroom spores are released from underneath the cap of the mushrooms (where there are typically gills, or pores). When a mushroom is mature enough, its spores will be released into the wild and are carried on the wind. Some of the spores will get lucky enough to land in a favorable environment where more mushrooms can be reproduced.

Many mushrooms will fruit on decomposing logs, in wet parts of the forest, or on trees. There are a few different kinds of spore-releasing that can happen when the mushrooms spread their spores. Some spores simply fall out of the mushroom and fly into the wind. Other mushrooms have a mechanism where they eject their spores out with more force. Spores will go on to create more mycelium, and mycelium, in turn, will fruit more mushrooms.

WHAT ARE MEDICINAL MUSHROOMS?

A "medicinal mushroom" is any mushroom that is safe for human consumption and has medicinal or health-enhancing properties. According to Professor Solomon P. Wasser, researcher at the University of Haifa and editor in chief of the *International Journal of Medicinal Mushrooms,* there are at least 650 species of mushrooms that are considered medicinal. You're going to meet 7 of the most well-researched mushrooms in this book. The great thing about the medicinal mushrooms in this book is that since they have always been completely legal (aside from psilocybin mushrooms), a lot of research has been done on them—with promising results for both everyday wellness concerns and serious conditions like cancer.

The mushrooms I've chosen to feature here in *The Rebel's Apothecary* have some of the most potent medicinal properties, including:

- Balancing the immune system
- Increasing energy and focus
- Calming the nervous system
- Soothing inflammation

- Providing antioxidants
- Exhibiting neuroprotective
  and neuroregenerative properties
- Stabilizing blood sugar
- Fighting cancer

As you'll see, these mushrooms can be *powerful* tools to have in your own personal healing toolbox.

Some of the medicinal mushrooms we'll cover in this book are great culinary mushrooms, too—meaning you can cook and eat them, just as you would with the mushrooms you're familiar with buying at the grocery store. In fact, one of the easiest ways to get more mushroom medicine into your life is to eat more of them. If you're one of those people who thinks they don't like mushrooms, I'm willing to bet it's because you haven't tried the ones that you'll soon end up loving! If you're basing your opinion of edible mushrooms on the raw mushrooms you typically see at salad bars, please forget about those and commit to giving a couple of different medicinal culinary mushrooms a try. Just wait until you stir-fry some shiitake or maitake mushrooms, or grill up some lion's mane—you'll become a mycophile (or "lover of mushrooms") in no time.

THE MEDICINE INSIDE THE MUSHROOMS

So what exactly are the compounds inside mushrooms that have proven to be so medicinal? Although each kind of medicinal mushroom has its own unique chemical makeup, they all contain types of polysaccharides known as beta-glucans, which have been shown to have immune-modulating and antitumor properties. Medicinal mushrooms also contain compounds called triterpenes, metabolites, and enzymes—all of which contribute to the power of mushrooms to support the immune system and nervous system, lower inflammation, and contribute to our energy, focus, and vitality.

In addition, each mushroom contains its own active medicinal compounds. For instance, turkey tail mushrooms contain a polysaccharide called PSK, cordyceps mushroom contains cordycepin, reishi contains triterpenes called ganoderic acids, and wild-harvested chaga contains powerful compounds called betulin and betulinic acid.

EACH MUSHROOM BRINGS US A UNIQUE MEDICINE.

"MUSHROOMS ARE ROCK STARS FOR OUR IMMUNE SYSTEMS, BUT THEY SUPPORT OTHER AREAS OF THE BODY TOO—LIKE THE NERVOUS SYSTEM, LIVER, CARDIOVASCULAR SYSTEM AND MORE. THEY ARE MORE NORMALIZING THAN STIMULATING—YOU CAN THINK OF THEM AS GENTLE IMMUNE TONICS," SAYS AVIVA ROMM, MD, AN INTEGRATIVE PHYSICIAN, MIDWIFE, AND HERBALIST WHO USES MEDICINAL MUSHROOMS IN HER PRACTICE.

EXTRACTING THE MEDICINE FROM MUSHROOMS

Medicinal mushrooms contain some compounds that can be extracted with water (beta-glucans and enzymes) and some that need to be extracted in alcohol (triterpenes). While each process can bring out beneficial compounds, both are needed to get the full array of medicine out of most mushrooms. When mushroom products are extracted for supplements, ideally they should go through a double-extraction process (usually in both hot water and alcohol) in order to extract all of the most beneficial compounds. Although there are some mushroom extracts and supplements on the market that are double-extracted, others aren't—so it's worth checking with the company or mushroom grower you're purchasing mushroom extracts from to make sure the product you're buying offers as many medicinal benefits as possible. Some of my favorite medicinal mushroom brands are listed in the Resources section.

MEDICINAL MUSHROOMS VS. MAGIC MUSHROOMS

The most common question I get when I start talking about medicinal mushrooms is, "Do you mean . . . *magic* mushrooms?" People automatically assume I'm talking about mushrooms with psychedelic effects, but that is not the case. The medicinal mushrooms you'll meet here aren't going to take you on a psychedelic journey, and they won't make you feel high. Many people consider psychedelic mushrooms, specifically psilocybin mushrooms, to be medicinal as well, and they absolutely can be. They have their very own healing properties, which you'll learn about soon.

THE SCIENTIFIC NAMES OF THE MUSHROOMS

You'll notice that in each mushroom section, I've included the scientific name along with the common name of each mushroom. Scientific names of plants and fungi are often used because they're the same across all languages, and are used by scientists and professionals in all published scientific research. They're also fun to learn. You can even make flash cards to memorize them if you want to (I did). Common names for mushrooms often differ from one region of the world to another, but the scientific names are standardized—which makes it easier to find, read, and understand clinical studies and research papers on medicinal mushrooms.

The seven medicinal mushrooms we'll be focusing on in *The Rebel's Apothecary* (and examples of their corresponding scientific names) are:

- **Chaga:** *Inonotus obliquus*

- **Reishi:** *Ganoderma lucidum, Ganoderma tsugae*

- **Lion's mane:** *Hericium erinaceus*

- **Cordyceps:** *Cordyceps sinensis, Cordyceps militaris*

- **Maitake:** *Grifola frondosa*

- **Shiitake:** *Lentinula edodes*

- **Turkey tail:** *Trametes versicolor*

There are many different classifications of mushrooms and different varieties of each species—but the names above are some of the most common.

HOW TO CONSUME MEDICINAL MUSHROOMS

When you start to dip your toe into the medicinal mushroom world, you'll see a vast array of mushroom products available.

Some of the ways to consume medicinal mushrooms are:

- Tinctures
- Extracts
- Powders

- Capsules

- Dried mushrooms

- Fresh mushrooms

- Teas

- Mushrooms infused into foods or beverages

There's a wide variety of ways to bring more healing mushrooms into your life, and you'll find recipes and usage suggestions sprinkled throughout the book.

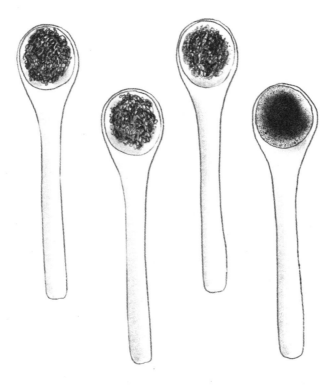

WHERE TO FIND MEDICINAL MUSHROOMS

Mushroom tinctures, extracts, powders, and capsules are available at health-food stores, online, and sometimes at farmer's markets if you have a local mushroom company where you live. My favorite way to purchase medicinal mushroom products is directly from the mushroom grower. I tend to buy my medicinal mushroom tinctures from the mycologists I've studied with, as I've watched them make their products and I know everything about their process. I've taken courses and gone on mushroom walks with both Tradd Cotter of Mushroom Mountain and John Michelotti of Catskill Fungi, and I feel confident about purchasing their products directly. If you have local mushroom companies in your area, they may sell products at your farmer's market or grocery store. To learn even more, sign up for a local mushroom class or take a mushroom walk led by an expert in your area. If that doesn't interest you and you just want to buy some mushrooms quickly, you can get great-quality medicinal mushroom products at health-food stores and online—but do your research to make sure the product has been double-extracted so you get as many healing benefits as possible. For double-extracted powders that you can mix into hot water, smoothies, or other beverages, I love the brands Four Sigmatic and SuperFeast. For more suggestions, see the Resources section.

For fresh culinary medicinal mushrooms, you'll want to start with your local grocery store or farmer's market, where you might find some of the edible mushrooms in this book (shiitake, maitake, and lion's mane). If you find fresh medicinal mushrooms at the farmer's market, talk to the mushroom farmers to see which mushrooms they love and ask how they cook them. Try new mushrooms one by one. Find your favorites! If you're shopping at a grocery store for your mushrooms, you might have luck finding the medicinal ones at a gourmet or specialty store. At many grocery stores, you're likely to find only the more common mushrooms—buttons, creminis, and portobellos—which are arguably the least medicinal mushrooms to eat but the easiest to find. Some of the medicinal mushrooms in this book (chaga and reishi, for example) aren't common at grocery stores, but a local herb shop may carry them.

CHOOSING MUSHROOM PRODUCTS: FRUITING BODY VS. MYCELIUM

When you head into a store or start searching online for a medicinal mushroom product, you'll find products that come from the fruiting bodies, products that come from the mycelium, and some that contain both. Since the fruiting body of the mushroom is made of highly condensed mycelium, it might make sense to assume that the fruiting body is going to be more potent with medicinal compounds, and most research points this way. There are different schools of thought about this, however; both fruiting-body extracts and mycelium extracts can be supportive for health.

The controversy arises from the fact that the mushroom mycelium in mycelium-based products is typically grown on grain substrates, and some products (powders and capsules, for instance) can contain large amounts of grain in them along with the mycelium. For this reason, many experts are proponents of products made with the fruiting body only—to avoid grain filler. Your product should say on the label whether it comes from fruiting bodies or mycelium, and if you can't figure it out, get in touch with the company and ask. The reputable, high-quality mushroom supplement companies will be transparent about their processes and happy to share those details with you.

While doing research for this book, I came across some mycologists and mushroom companies that use fruiting bodies only, and others that use mycelium. There are proponents for both, however, most of the published studies show that fruiting bodies have higher concentrations of beneficial constituents.

On their website, the popular mushroom beverage extract brand Four Sigmatic shares about their choice to use fruiting bodies to make their mushroom extracts:

"We do agree that all parts of the fungi have their benefits, however we choose to use the fruiting bodies of mushrooms, and never mycelium grown on grains. Normally, mycelium based products contain 50–80% starch from the growing substrate, up to 50% less beta-glucans than fruiting bodies, and far less beneficial compounds."

Paul Stamets, who owns another of the most popular medicinal mushroom supplement companies, Host Defense, is an advocate for the benefits of mycelium.

"Mushroom mycelium is an excellent ingredient for supporting health," Stamets says. "When produced and processed properly, mushroom mycelium contains a vast range of compounds, including enzymes, prebiotics, antioxidants, and polysaccharides to support immunity."

Regarding the fruiting body vs. mycelium question, Robert Rogers, author of *The Fungal Pharmacy,* has said, "It would appear both fruiting bodies and mycelium have much to offer. I consume both, the latter as powder in vegetable and fruit smoothies in the morning and the former in tincture or extract form, when I feel the need."

By all accounts, there are numerous benefits to using both fruiting bodies and mycelium. The mushroom products I personally take on a daily basis primarily come from the fruiting bodies, although I do experiment with mycelium products as well. Your best bet would be to try the mushroom product you feel most drawn to, take it for a few weeks, and see how you feel.

COOKED VS. RAW MUSHROOMS

Although we're going to be focused on medicinal mushrooms in this book, I want to cover a couple of general mushroom questions that I get a lot—questions that I had myself before doing this research—about the most common mushrooms you're probably familiar with. When I think of a raw mushroom, I picture a salad bar with sliced white button mushrooms. Top those babies with ranch dressing and some iceberg lettuce, and you're good to go. At least, that's what I thought of as mushrooms for most of my life. Does anyone actually find it appetizing to eat mushrooms this way? After you experience cooking with the more medicinal mushrooms (especially when you make them with butter and garlic!), you'll never want to go back to eating raw, chalky-textured mushrooms from a salad bar again. In fact, most experts recommend not eating mushrooms raw at all.

Mushrooms have a tough cell wall called chitin that our digestive systems can't break down, and in order to release the nutrients in the mushrooms, they must be cooked well. In addition, there may be even more important reasons to cook mushrooms rather than eating them raw.

Something that blew my mind when I first started learning about mushrooms is that button mushrooms, creminis, or "baby bellas," and portobellos are all the same species—*Agaricus bisporus*. White buttons and creminis are the same exact species, just a different color (similar to a white or brown eggshell). Portobellos are older versions of these mushrooms that have had more time to mature, and their caps have opened up. So when you see buttons, creminis, and portobellos as the only three options at the store, well, they're all actually *the same mushroom*. Isn't that wild? But these seemingly innocent mushrooms may, in fact, be the least medicinal mushrooms you can eat, especially when they're raw.

As it turns out, some raw mushrooms contain a potentially carcinogenic compound called agaritine—this compound is present in buttons, creminis, and portobellos. The agaritine needs to be cooked out of these mushrooms, which is why it's recommended to cook them well before consuming. There is some debate over how much of a concern this should be, but based on nutrient availability alone, I say skip the raw mushrooms at the salad bar (you're welcome!) and always opt for cooked.

Dr. Andrew Weil has said, "In general, I advise against eating a lot of the familiar cultivated white or 'button' mushrooms found on supermarket shelves throughout the United States. They are among a number of foods that contain natural carcinogens. We don't know how dangerous these toxins are, but we do know that they do not occur in other mushrooms that offer great health benefits. If you're going to eat them, cook them well, at high temperatures, by sautéing, broiling, or grilling. Heat breaks down many of the toxic constituents."

CHOOSING ORGANIC MUSHROOMS

Mushrooms are bioaccumulators (so is cannabis!), which means they will highly absorb whatever is in the soil (such as heavy metals and pesticides). This means you should choose organically grown or certified naturally grown mushrooms and mushroom supplements whenever possible. Of course, some small companies are growing high-quality mushrooms and using organic practices but haven't yet obtained organic certification—so talk to your local mushroom grower about their process. I've found mushroom growers (and mushroom enthusiasts in general) to be the friendliest of people, and they will be happy to share their mushroom love with you.

WHY SOME MUSHROOMS ARE SO EXPENSIVE

The first time I started scouting the grocery stores for new mushrooms to try, I had sticker shock when I saw the chanterelles. Forty-four dollars per pound? Why are these chanterelle mushrooms so expensive, when the oyster mushrooms right next to them are selling for only six dollars per pound?

When you find a grocery store that has a wide variety of mushrooms, you'll likely see some that have a much higher price than the others. This is because some mushrooms can't be cultivated—they can be found only in the wild. These mushrooms are known as mycorrhizal mushrooms, which means they have a symbiotic relationship with a particular type of tree or soil—they only grow in specific places at specific times of year, and we haven't figured out how to reliably cultivate them commercially. These mycorrhizal beauties are highly coveted by mycophiles, and are prized with great enthusiasm when found on foraging trips.

On the flip side, some mushrooms can be easily cultivated on mushroom farms, or even at home, and therefore these mushrooms tend to be less expensive when you find them at the store.

A few examples of mushrooms that can be cultivated are oysters, shiitakes, maitakes, lion's mane, and the "grocery-store mushrooms"—buttons, creminis, and portobellos. A few examples of mycorrhizal mushrooms that can be grown only in the wild are chanterelles, morels, truffles, and porcinis.

MUSHROOM FORAGING IN THE WILD

As you deepen your knowledge of the many wondrous properties of mushrooms, you're likely going to want to go find some for yourself. If you do have the urge to go mushroom foraging in the wild, I encourage you to join your local mycological society and find out when the group is doing a guided mushroom walk, or "foray." You'll want to go with experienced foragers, because there are some look-alike mushrooms out there—species that may be harmful or poisonous, but look similar to edible mushrooms. Don't go out into the woods alone and try to identify and eat your own edible mushrooms—make sure you go with an experienced guide. If you do find yourself foraging, I've learned from my herbalist teachers that anytime you're picking something in the wild, it's best not to take more than one-third of whatever presents itself. You don't want to completely eliminate a patch of anything—this goes for foraging all herbs, plants, and mushrooms. If you're inspired to grow your own medicinal mushrooms, there are some great companies that offer home growing kits. I recently purchased one for my dad from a company called North Spore.

DOSING WITH MEDICINAL MUSHROOMS

Each producer of mushroom supplements will have their own dose listed on the label. These recommendations are typically pretty conservative, so the label's dose can be a good place to start. However, when it comes to dosing with medicinal mushrooms—just like cannabis—there isn't a "one-size-fits-all" dose that works for everyone.

The good news is that all of the mushrooms you'll learn about next are considered safe and nontoxic, as long as you're getting a good mushroom product from a quality source.

If you're looking to medicinal mushrooms for daily wellness, the general recommended starting dose (in extract form—which means powders, capsules, or tinctures) is about 1000–3000 mg (1–3 grams) per day. This will typically be something like 2 capsules, 1–2 dropperfuls of a tincture, or 1–2 teaspoons of powder extract.

If you're using medicinal mushrooms to treat a more serious condition, a higher dose may be more effective.

"With medicinal mushrooms, there's a maintenance dose and a condition dose," said mycologist Tradd Cotter at a seminar I attended at his South Carolina research facility, Mushroom Mountain. "One dried gram or five fresh grams of mushrooms is a typical maintenance dose for a 160-pound adult. A condition dose (if you have cancer, for example) is usually about five times the amount of a maintenance dose."

These dosing guidelines are general, as each product, person, and condition are different.

Of course, when you're taking a high dose of any herb or supplement, do so under the guidance of your healthcare professional, and make sure there are no potential interactions with medications you're taking. Memorial Sloan Kettering Cancer Center has a fantastic website that lists potential drug interactions with many different common herbs, mushrooms, and dietary supplements.

> ### MEDICINAL MUSHROOM DOSING QUICK GUIDE
>
> - Typical dose for daily wellness/maintenance: 1000–3000 mg (1–3 g) per day
> - About 2 capsules, 1–2 dropperfuls of a tincture, or 1–2 teaspoons of powder extract
> - Typical condition dose: 3000–10,000 mg (3–10 g) per day
> - Calculate dosage based on the label of the product you choose
>
> *These are only very general guidelines. Start with a daily mainte-nance dose, monitor any effects you feel, and work under the guidance of your healthcare practitioner.*

Now, let's dive in to the healing properties of seven of the most po-tent medicinal mushrooms.

CHAGA (*INONOTUS OBLIQUUS*)

IMMUNITY, DETOXIFYING, ANTI-INFLAMMATORY

Chaga is often referred to as the "king" of the medicinal mushrooms, with good reason. Chaga has been shown to balance the immune system, reduce inflammation, and provide a high level of antioxidants, making it one of the best overall wellness mushrooms. When chaga's medicine is extracted through double extraction (with both hot water and alco-hol), it has been shown to have antiviral and antitumor properties.

Chaga isn't one of the edible mushrooms, which means you can't just

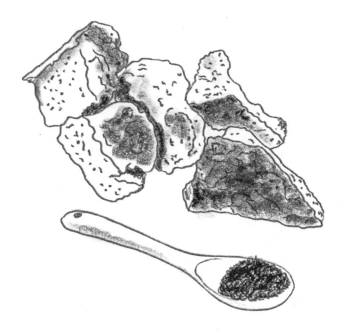

take chaga as you'd find it in the wild and eat it. You can, however, find its potent detoxifying powers extracted into teas, powders, tinctures, and capsules. Chaga looks like a caramel-brown piece of cork with a hard black coating around it. Chaga grows on birch trees, and acts as a parasite to the birch tree it inhabits. Even though chaga may be parasitic to the birch tree, it offers tremendous health benefits to us as humans. Chaga is an ancient, wild mushroom that grows naturally in cold north-ern climates (Siberia, Poland, and Canada, for example), and many be-lieve that chaga's harsh-weather resilience is part of the reason it can help us fight infections and viruses, and generally boost our immune health.

When I first learned of my dad's cancer diagnosis, one of the first people I called was my friend David "Avocado" Wolfe. I knew that as a superfood and wild-food nutrition expert (and one of the first people who inspired me to study holistic nutrition), he'd have an opinion on a supplement or herb I could look into to support my dad during chemotherapy. I had a feeling David Avocado would steer me toward medicinal mushrooms—and, of course, he did.

"Chaga extracted in alcohol is one of the most potent tumor-fighting compounds I've ever seen," he said. He feels so strongly about chaga that he dedicated a whole book to it (appropriately named *Chaga: King of the Medicinal Mushrooms*). That sentence stuck with me, and I found the research to back it up. In Russia, they have been using chaga extracts in alcohol tinctures as a cancer therapy for decades, and studies show antitumor activity on various kinds of cancer cells with chaga—this includes water extracts, alcohol extracts, and mycelium extracts.

Once I started researching the ins and outs of chaga, I learned that it's absolutely packed with vitamins, minerals, and antioxidants. In fact, it's one of the highest-antioxidant foods in the world, right up there with cacao.

The antioxidants and beta-glucans inside chaga give it incredible immune system–balancing properties. Chaga is immunomodulating, which means it acts as an adaptogen for the immune system—if your immune system is either overactive or underactive, chaga can help to bring it back into balance so your body can go back to its regularly scheduled program of fighting infections and maintaining homeostasis in the body. It's a great mushroom to take if you feel like you might be coming down with a cold.

Chaga's benefits:

- Anti-inflammatory
- High in antioxidants

- Immune balancing
- Antiviral
- Antitumor
- Soothes digestion
- Stabilizes blood sugar
- Soothes skin

Chaga is a truly "foundational" medicine, in the sense that you can use it regularly to support a baseline level of good health, as well as using it more potently when you're working to support the healing of a more serious condition.

One of the most popular ways to consume chaga is by making tea, and as you read on, you'll find a recipe. In fact, chaga was used as a coffee substitute in Russia during World War II, as there were strict coffee rations—but chaga was found in abundance. I frequently make chaga tea at home from either a piece of chaga or chaga powder. Sipping a mug of hot chaga tea feels like being enveloped in a warm, earthy hug. It has hints of vanilla flavor due to the vanillin that's inside it (the same compound in vanilla), which makes it perfect for tea.

Sustainability of Chaga Harvesting

Because chaga shows up on approximately only 1 in every 10,000 birch trees, there are concerns about sustainability. Chaga is one of the fungi that is not easily cultivated—the majority of chaga sold is wild-harvested (although there are some who have been able to produce cultivated chaga mycelium that doesn't come from birch trees). However, some of the most potent medicinal properties of chaga are due to the betulin content, which comes directly from birch bark, so wild-harvested chaga is considered to be medicinally superior.

If you find yourself foraging for chaga out in the wild, one of the most important things you can do is not take the entire chunk of chaga from the tree. You want to honor the tree and the forest, and leave enough so it can grow back. If you're purchasing wild-harvested chaga, find out if the company you're purchasing from uses sustainable chaga-harvesting practices. A phone call or email to the company should be sufficient if they don't have information about their harvesting practices on their website.

How to Get Started with Chaga Mushrooms

- **Make tea.** You can find chunks of chaga at many health-food stores and herb shops, or online. Directions for making tea are coming up next. Bonus: If you're going to be simmering soup or broth for a long period of time, you can add a chunk of chaga to it and extract the medicinal benefits. Make sure to take it out before serving.

- **Use a double-extracted powder.** Chaga powder extracts are easy to stir into water, coffee, tea, or a smoothie. You can find chaga in capsules as well, but you'll be missing out on that awesome chaga taste.

- **Take a tincture.** There are beneficial compounds in chaga (such as betulinic acid) that don't get extracted by water alone—some of these compounds need to be extracted in alcohol. I keep a chaga tincture on my kitchen counter, and sometimes I'll add a dropperful of the tincture to my homemade chaga tea (tea is a water extraction), for more potent benefits. You can find some wonderful chaga tinctures online or at your local health-food store—or make your own at home! John Michelotti from Catskill Fungi has shared his chaga tincture recipe with us, on page 165.

Chaga Tea

It takes just a tiny piece of chaga to make a big pot of chaga tea, and it's one of my favorite wellness rituals. I drink it hot when I first make it, and then move it into the fridge to have iced chaga tea for a couple of days. You can use chaga tea as a base for smoothies, you can add it into your French press instead of water to make your coffee, and you can even freeze chaga tea to make chaga ice cubes.

This is a great tea to make if you're feeling under the weather or want to soothe your digestion. Chaga tea doesn't contain caffeine (in fact, no mushrooms contain caffeine!), so you can drink it morning or night.

Makes 8 cups of tea

To make an earthy, potent, smooth, and medicinal chaga tea, you'll need:

1 small chunk of chaga (about 1 inch)

8 cups water

In a large pot, simmer water and chaga for at minimum 20 minutes (at least 1 hour is ideal for extracting the medicine), or as long as 5 hours, with the top on. Add more water if the water starts to evaporate. The longer you boil it, the more potent your chaga tea will be. When it's ready, you'll have a dark, rich tea.

Remove the chaga and pour the liquid into a mug. Sip.

You can also reuse your piece of chaga 2–3 more times after the initial brew—you'll know it's time to stop using it when the water doesn't turn dark brown anymore. After you make tea, you can use your chaga chunk to make an alcohol tincture if desired.

You can add your favorite sweetener (such as a touch of raw honey, maple syrup, or stevia), and your milk of choice—but I prefer it natural.

REISHI (GANODERMA LUCIDUM)

ANTI-STRESS, LONGEVITY, IMMUNITY

When I said chaga is the king of mushrooms, I bet you were wondering, "Who's the queen?" Enter reishi. Reishi is known as the queen of mushrooms, the mushroom of immortality, the mushroom of spiritual potency, or the lingzhi mushroom. It's one of the most prized mushrooms in traditional Chinese medicine and has been used medicinally for more than 2,000 years in China and Japan. Reishi gets its nickname—"mushroom of immortality"—because it's widely known as the most powerful mushroom for longevity.

Reishi is a potent anti-inflammatory mushroom, and it is often used for lowering stress and helping to soothe the nervous system. It's

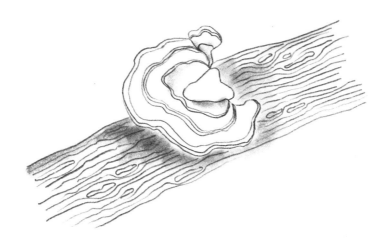

a great mushroom to take at night, or any time you want to calm your nerves and get back into balance.

As with chaga, reishi isn't directly edible—it's a very hard mushroom, with a shiny red outer cap—but it's wonderful in teas and extracts. I often make reishi tea when I'm winding down to get ready to sleep, and I travel with packets of reishi extract powder to keep my immune system strong and to help me stay relaxed and grounded. I've made reishi tea many times in hotel rooms, using a powdered reishi extract and the hot water from the in-room coffeemaker—there's nothing more comfy than snuggling under a blanket at night with a hot mug of reishi tea in the winter. If you have both chaga and reishi tea on rotation in your home, well, consider yourself cloaked in mushroom royalty.

Reishi is one of the most widely studied mushrooms, is one of the most powerful mushrooms for immunity, and is commonly used as an adjunct to traditional cancer treatments. A 2012 study by Dr. Solomon Wasser showed that the ganoderic acid from both reishi fruiting bodies and mycelium demonstrated antitumor and immunomodulating activity, inducing apoptosis (cell death) of cancer cells.

Reishi has been shown to protect DNA from oxidative stress, and it has a high level of antioxidants, which can fight free radicals in the body—and keep skin healthy, too. Reishi has also been shown to help with histamine response, so it's a great mushroom to take if you commonly suffer from seasonal allergies. It has also been shown to help regulate blood sugar.

In short, reishi is a medicinal mushroom powerhouse.

"Every day, I take chaga, lion's mane, and reishi—but if I could only take one, I'd choose reishi," says John Michelotti of Catskill Fungi. "Reishi is great for my seasonal allergies, supporting my immune system, and helps to balance my energy levels and relax my nervous system."

Some of reishi's healing benefits:

- Lowers stress and calms nervous system
- Improves sleep quality
- Helps with seasonal allergies
- Balances the immune system
- Promotes longevity
- Regulates blood sugar
- Promotes healthy liver function
- Can inhibit tumor growth

How to Get Started with Reishi Mushrooms

- **Make tea.** Reishi is another mushroom that's great for making tea. You can find dried reishi at many health-food stores or herb stores and online. You'll want to make reishi tea in a similar manner as you'd make chaga tea—simmer the dried reishi in hot water for 30 minutes to 2 hours—the longer the better, as far as extracting the benefits goes, but the longer you simmer it, the more bitter-tasting your tea will be. Because reishi has a stronger, more bitter taste than chaga, some people prefer adding a sweetener such as honey or stevia to reishi tea. I like to drink down the bitterness, though—I tend to like the taste of medicinal herbs. Herbalist often say that tasting the herbs alerts the body that medicine is coming. Of course, as a quicker version of this tea, you can use an extracted reishi mushroom powder to stir into hot water.

- **Add a piece of dried reishi to soups or stews while cooking.** If you can find dried reishi at your local herb shop, you can add it to your soups, stews, or broths while cooking, and remove the piece of reishi before eating. This infuses reishi's water-soluble compounds into your meal, which can help boost immunity. This is an easy trick to rely on during the cold season, or whenever your vitality could use a little boost. (Bonus: Add both chaga and reishi!)

- **Take a double-extracted powder.** You can also find dried reishi powders that have been double-extracted (I like Four Sigmatic or SuperFeast) to get all of the beneficial medicine. This can be stirred into water, tea, coffee, or smoothies or taken as a capsule.

- **Take a tincture.** Like chaga, reishi has compounds in it that need to be alcohol-extracted, so the tea won't deliver all of the beneficial properties on its own. Alcohol tinctures are a great way to get all of the medicinal compounds out of the reishi mushroom. My favorite tinctures are from Catskill Fungi and MycoMatrix.

LION'S MANE (*HERICIUM ERINACEUS*)

BRAIN HEALTH, MENTAL FOCUS, NERVE SUPPORT

Lion's mane is a fascinating-looking mushroom that gets its name from its fuzzy and furry natural appearance—it actually looks like a lion's mane! My deep dive into using lion's mane mushrooms began with Tim Ferriss's podcast episode with Paul Stamets (episode 340 of *The Tim Ferriss Show*). I was already familiar with lion's mane for focus and concentration, and I had been taking it myself in powdered extract form—usually before sitting down to work or write. I would sprinkle lion's mane powder into my coffee, tea, or smoothies, and I also had

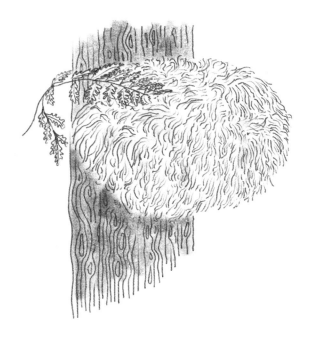

lion's mane capsules on hand. Although the brain-boosting properties I experienced from taking lion's mane were subtle, whenever I took it I felt more clear, focused, and able to put my thoughts onto paper in a much more streamlined way than without lion's mane.

While listening to that podcast episode, however, my interest in lion's mane deepened. Tim and Paul discussed the neuroregenerative properties of lion's mane—that it's promising for repairing the myelin sheath around damaged nerves and can be helpful for brain and nerve conditions such as Alzheimer's, dementia, Parkinson's, and neuropathy. You can think of the myelin sheath around nerves as the protective coating around an electrical wire—if the coating breaks down, the wire is exposed. Lion's mane can help to regenerate that protective coating around our nerves.

After hearing this, my further research revealed positive testimonials about lion's mane helping to improve a wide range of conditions. Nerve pain decreasing. Nerve damage improving. Brain fog eliminated. More mental clarity. Sharper memory. Feeling clear minded and creative. People were reporting improvements in all of these areas, and for me, there was enough anecdotal evidence to warrant a lion's mane experiment.

At the time, my dad was about a year into his chemotherapy treatments, and the only side effect I'd heard him complain about was neuropathy—he often felt a tingling sensation in his fingers and toes. I asked my dad if he'd be willing to add another mushroom to his daily routine, and he was willing to try it.

Two weeks after beginning a regimen of taking two lion's mane capsules every day, my dad reported that he could now "feel the difference between a dime and a quarter in his pocket" with the tips of his fingers, which hadn't been the case before taking the lion's mane. He was also able to feel his contact lenses on his fingertips again, which he had lost the ability to do. His oncologist had warned him that he may begin to have trouble typing on a keyboard and buttoning buttons due to the chemo drugs—but since starting with the lion's mane, his neuropathy has gotten better instead of worse.

A 2013 study in the *International Journal of Medicinal Mushrooms* showed that lion's mane contains active compounds that stimulate nerve growth factor (NGF). The deterioration of NGF is related to Alzheimer's disease and dementia, which suggests, as Paul Stamets noted in the podcast episode, that lion's mane could be a helpful preventative for cognitive decline. No toxic or negative side effects have been reported from taking lion's mane.

To summarize, lion's mane mushroom can promote:

- Improved memory
- Enhanced clarity, creativity, and focus
- Neuro-protective properties
- Repairing of nerve damage or relief of nerve pain/neuropathy
- Improved cognitive function and brain health
- Improved mood

One of the greatest things about lion's mane is that it's a medicinal mushroom you can cook and eat. Lion's mane mushrooms are sometimes used as a meat substitute because of their texture, which is a bit like the texture of lobster or crab. I often find lion's mane mushrooms at my local farmer's market, and I'm always thrilled when I do. If you find fresh lion's mane, don't be intimidated—they're very easy to cook.

Lion's mane is one of the easiest mushrooms to cultivate, and you can even grow your own at home (I've ordered lion's mane growing kits from a company called North Spore).

How to Get Started with Lion's Mane Mushrooms

- **Eat them.** Eating lion's mane may not be the most potent way to get as much medicine from them as possible (it's much more condensed in an extract), but they're delicious. Because of their fuzziness, it's not recommended that you wash them unless there's a lot of dirt on them that you can't brush off. If you do wash them, be sure to dry them well before you cook them—they hold a lot of water and will take much longer to cook if they're wet. To keep it simple, slice them up and sauté them in a pan with butter until they're toasty and browned. To take your lion's mane cooking to the next level, make sure to try Chef Seamus Mullen's recipe, Lion's Mane Braised in Coconut, on page 157— it's incredible.

- **Take a tincture.** I've been experimenting with different forms of lion's mane mushroom for a few years now, and I can feel the effects the most strongly when I take it in a tincture. I put it directly on my tongue and wash it down with water, or add it to water or tea before I sit down to write or research, which helps me to feel sharper and clearer.

- **Use a powder extract.** Lion's mane comes as a powder extract, too. I use powder extracts fairly often, especially for traveling— they're great to add to coffee, tea, hot water, or a smoothie. If you're the kind of person who prefers to consume capsules due to the convenience and simplicity, you can find those, too. My dad has had great success with his neuropathy by taking lion's mane capsules.

CORDYCEPS (*CORDYCEPS SINENSIS/MILITARIS*)

ENERGY, STAMINA, ADRENAL SUPPORT

I've always gravitated toward foods and supplements that claim to help with energy—so when I heard cordyceps was the go-to mushroom for energy and stamina, it immediately took the seat at the head of my table. The first time I tried cordyceps mushrooms was in powdered extract form, and I mixed it into my coffee. What I noticed right off the bat was that the energy I usually get from coffee seemed to last longer—instead of a quick spike, I felt a more balanced energy. I was curious to see what cordyceps would be like on its own, so the next time

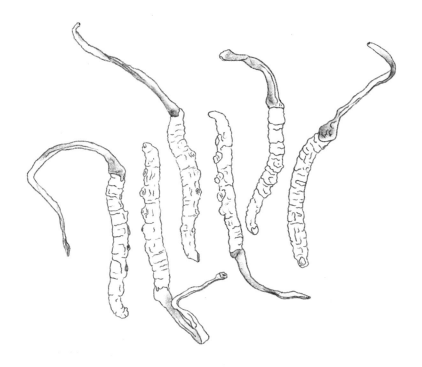

I tried it, I put a packet of cordyceps mushroom powder into hot water. Drinking cordyceps tea gave me an energy boost in the afternoon without any jitteriness or crash—I just felt uplifted. I've also found it to be a great pick-me-up to take before a workout or yoga class.

Cordyceps is the star mushroom for energy and adrenal support. Studies have shown that cordyceps mushroom reduces fatigue and can improve endurance, oxygen uptake, and athletic performance.

Cordyceps enhances our energy by increasing adenosine triphosphate (ATP) in our cells, which is essential for energy production. Traditionally, cordyceps has been used as an aphrodisiac—it's been shown to boost testosterone levels, increase sperm production, enhance libido (in both sexes), and improve blood circulation.

Cordyceps can help restore energy depleted by stress—in Japan, it's used to treat postpartum exhaustion.

And as if that wasn't enough, just like the other mushrooms we've met so far, cordyceps has anti-inflammatory, anticancer, and immune-modulating properties. Cordyceps is best taken in extract form—capsules, powder, or tincture.

As far as how it's cultivated, cordyceps is a bit of a weird one. Cordyceps mushrooms grow on *caterpillars*. That's right, these "caterpillar fungi" traditionally grow on the bodies of insects in the Himalayas, traditionally used in Tibet and Nepal. It's said that Nepalese cattle herders noticed that the cows grazing on cordyceps were gaining strength and reproductive capacity. The locals began to consume it and touted enhanced energy, vigor, and aphrodisiac effects.

But not to worry—humans have found ways to cultivate cordyceps without insects, so the cordyceps supplements you'll find at your local health-food store are caterpillar-free (and completely vegetarian). These cultivated varieties are known as *Cordyceps militaris,* rather than insect-grown (*Cordyceps sinensis*). While wild cultivated cordyceps is still available, mostly in Asia, it is very rare—and very expensive.

A few ways cordyceps can support you:

- Enhances energy and reduces fatigue
- Improves endurance, stamina, and athletic performance
- Elevates sex drive
- Helps the body better cope with stress
- Boosts mood
- Provides high levels of antioxidants

How to Get Started with Cordyceps Mushrooms

- **Use a double-extracted powder.** While it *is* possible to cook with the actual mushroom fruiting body and make teas with it, you aren't likely to find cordyceps in your grocery store, unless you live in Asia, where it can be found at local markets. An easy way to get started with the benefits of cordyceps is to use a powder extract—I often add cordyceps powder to coffee, tea, or hot water when I need a little boost. You can also add the powder to an energizing smoothie (try the Ultimate Aphrodisiac Smoothie recipe on page 234). Cordyceps powder works well in recipes, too—Olga Cotter of Mushroom Mountain shares her delicious Cordyceps Energy Bars recipe on page 219.

- **Take tincture or capsule.** Cordyceps can also be taken in liquid extract form as a tincture, or as a powder in capsules.

MAITAKE (*GRIFOLA FRONDOSA*)

BLOOD-SUGAR-STABILIZING, IMMUNITY

Maitake is another medicinal mushroom that will win your heart—not only because it's incredibly delicious to cook with (I like to sauté it in coconut oil or grass-fed butter with a little bit of flaky sea salt), but it has potent healing properties. Maitake is known as the dancing mushroom—some say this nickname comes from the

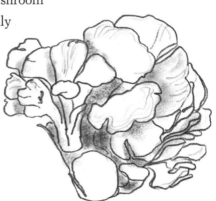

joy experienced by whoever has the good fortune of finding maitake growing under a tree. It's also called hen of the woods, as it resembles a hen! Maitake mushrooms are rich in antioxidants and beta-glucans, which make them a supportive mushroom to add to any wellness regimen. Maitake mushrooms have been found to balance blood sugar and improve insulin sensitivity, and for this reason, maitake has been used traditionally to help with diabetes and weight loss. Maitake can also help to lower cholesterol and blood pressure.

"I use maitake in my practice particularly for immune support, but also for my patients who have insulin resistance and metabolic syndrome, because it helps with blood pressure and blood sugar," says Aviva Romm, MD.

Just like the other mushrooms you've met so far, maitake has been shown to help with cancer treatment—slowing tumor growth and alleviating some of the side effects of chemotherapy by keeping the immune system strong.

The compound in maitake called D-fraction has been shown to help modulate the immune system and increase natural killer cells, which can help fight tumors. Studies have shown that maitake may be helpful in reducing breast, liver, and lung cancer tumors, and has been used in conjunction with chemotherapy treatments to enhance immune function.

Some of the main benefits of maitake:

- Immune system support
- Helps to balance blood sugar
- Can support weight loss
- Antitumor effects

- Supports healthy cholesterol levels

- Can lower blood pressure

- Anti-inflammatory and high in antioxidants

How to Get Started with Maitake Mushrooms

- **Eat them.** Maitake mushrooms are some of the most delicious edible medicinal mushrooms, and can be found at many grocery stores or at your local farmer's market. You'll want to break the bottom part off (the nub where the mushroom is attached), and use just the feathery parts of the mushroom for cooking. I typically cook maitake either by breaking apart the pieces and roasting them in the oven or by sautéing them in a pan with grass-fed butter or coconut oil until they're browned. You can add cooked maitake mushrooms to a salad or eggs, throw them into a stir-fry, add them to tacos, or sprinkle them with salt, pepper, fresh herbs, and a spritz of lemon juice and eat them straight out of a bowl. You can find a great, simple recipe for Grilled Maitake Mushrooms from my friend Chef Will Hickox on page 161.

- **Use tinctures, extract powders, or capsules.** I think cooking with maitake is the easiest way to add more of the "dancing mushroom" into your life, but if you want to get a potent, medicinal dose of maitake, you can find it in tinctures, extract powders, and capsules, available at health-food stores or online.

- **Make tea with dried maitakes.** When I was at Mushroom Mountain taking a seminar led by mycologist Tradd Cotter, he made Maitake Mint Tea for us (recipe on page 163), which was surprisingly delicious, considering maitake is a savory-tasting mushroom. You can find dried maitakes for tea online or at some health-food stores.

SHIITAKE (*LENTINULA EDODES*)

IMMUNITY, ANTIVIRAL

Of all the mushrooms in *The Rebel's Apothecary,* shiitakes are the ones most commonly found at grocery stores and on restaurant menus. In fact, shiitakes may be the only medicinal mushrooms you'll see in the grocery store aisle. Shiitake mushrooms are common in Asian cooking, and they are known for bringing out that rich, umami flavor in savory dishes.

If you love eating shiitake mushrooms like I do, you can probably imagine why I was so happy to find out that not only are they incredibly delicious, but they have plenty of healing benefits, too. If you eat shiitakes regularly, you've already been taking advantage of their healing magic.

Because shiitake mushrooms can be easily cultivated (not only wild

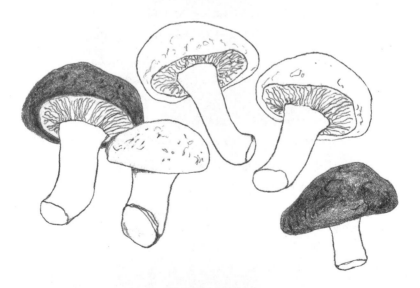

grown), they are available in abundance, and often at a lower price point than other gourmet/medicinal mushrooms.

Shiitake mushrooms have a whole host of medicinal benefits, so adding them into your diet or as a supplement can be a great way to support overall health. Studies have shown that eating shiitake mushrooms can improve immunity, lower cholesterol, and reduce inflammation in the body.

In Japan and China, the active compound in shiitake (lentinan) is commonly used in cancer treatment in conjunction with chemotherapy, as it's been shown to inhibit tumor growth, enhance the effectiveness of some chemotherapy drugs, and prevent damage to the immune system during treatment. One of the first supplements I started researching when my dad got cancer is called active hexose correlated compound (AHCC), which is a supplement made primarily from the mycelium of shiitake mushrooms. Multiple studies have shown that AHCC can be effective in reducing side effects of chemotherapy drugs and improving immune response in patients with chemotherapy-weakened immune systems. My dad has been taking it for over two years, along with chemotherapy, and his immune system has remained very strong. While I'm not claiming direct cause and effect (the strength of his health could be attributed to *many* things), after reviewing the research, I think it's safe to say the AHCC from shiitake mushrooms could be helping.

Shiitake has also been shown to have potent antiviral effects. Studies have shown success in people using AHCC to combat human papillomavirus (HPV) and the flu virus. In a recent clinical trial, 60 percent of HPV patients taking 3 g of AHCC per day showed no sign of infection after six months.

"One of the best antivirals comes from shiitake," says mycologist

Tradd Cotter. "Shiitakes are widely available and affordable. During flu season, take a shiitake tincture, and eat more shiitakes."

Shiitakes are some of the most promising mushrooms to add to your apothecary—namely, because they're so easy to find, are inexpensive, and have extremely promising health benefits.

Some of the medicinal properties of shiitake:

- Immune system support

- Antiviral properties

- Antitumor properties

- Can lower blood pressure and cholesterol

- Supports healthy skin

- Anti-inflammatory

How to Get Started with Shiitake Mushrooms

- **Eat them.** Shiitake, just like maitake, is a delicious edible mushroom that can be used in so many ways—in soups, stews, or stir-fries, sautéed, baked, added to eggs, or in a salad. Try substituting shiitakes for any other mushroom you typically cook with, or any recipe that calls for mushrooms. Shiitake "bacon" is one of my favorite things to make—I slice shiitakes up into thin strips and bake them in the oven or sauté them in a pan until crispy (Shiitake or Maitake Bacon recipe on page 154). I've also swapped shiitakes into my favorite mushroom gravy recipe, where I used to use creminis (the Shiitake Gravy recipe is on page 160). The possibilities are virtually endless when it comes to what you can do with shiitakes!

- **Take them as AHCC capsules.** If you're hoping to support your immune system during chemotherapy or any other time when your immune function may be compromised, you may want to try AHCC capsules. There's a lot of research into AHCC for the immune system, and in Japan AHCC is the second-most-widely-used supplement by cancer patients. (*Agaricus blazei,* another medicinal mushroom, is number one.)

- **Tinctures, powder extracts, or capsules.** Just like the other mushrooms mentioned, you can take shiitake in many different forms, depending on your preference. Shiitake mushrooms are available as tinctures, powder extracts, or capsules. The tinctures and capsules can be taken orally, and the powder extracts can be stirred into food or drink—like teas, broths, and soups.

TURKEY TAIL (*TRAMETES VERSICOLOR*)

IMMUNITY, ANTIVIRAL, ANTITUMOR

Turkey tail was one of the first medicinal mushrooms I got ac-quainted with (and fast!) when I found out about my dad's can-cer diagnosis. The compounding pharmacist at Dr. Frank Lipman's functional medicine practice suggested I look into it as an adjunct to chemotherapy. As it turns out, it's known to be a tumor-fighting mushroom that can also provide robust immune system support, which is useful not only for cancer patients but for general wellness and disease prevention too.

Turkey tail mushroom has been studied for its antitumor effects (particularly on breast cancer, but it's been shown to have antitumor effects in other types of cancer as well), and has been used in traditional Chinese medicine for immune system support for thousands of years. It's also been shown to help chemotherapy and radiation become more effective for some patients, and is considered to be anti-inflammatory and immune system–modulating. Krestin, a drug derived from the PSK (polysaccharide-K) in turkey tail mushrooms, has been an officially approved cancer treatment in Japan since 1977.

"Turkey tail has been used in Asia for thousands and thousands of years, and it turns out to be a really potent immune therapy," says Dr. Leanna J. Standish, medical director of the Bastyr Integrative Oncology Research Center.

In a 2011 TEDMED talk, Paul Stamets described how his mother healed from stage IV breast cancer with the help of turkey tail mushrooms. His story is compelling and helped to support my research on turkey tail for cancer. "Take these mushrooms as an adjunct therapy—not as a substitution—but to support the immune system. Natural killer cells increase on a dose-dependent basis," he says in the talk. A study of women with breast cancer found that participants who took between 6 and 9 grams of turkey tail powder extract per day experienced an increase in cancer-fighting cells in the immune system (natural killer cells and lymphocytes).

According to the Memorial Sloan Kettering Cancer Center, PSK and PSP, the polysaccharide compounds in turkey tail, have also shown promise in fighting viruses, including HIV and herpes.

If you're fortunate enough to see turkey tail in the wild, you'll understand immediately where it got its name. It most commonly grows on decomposing logs in the forest, and the rings of color that line the mushroom, along with the fanlike shape, make it look just like the tail of a turkey. I came across it on one of my mushroom walks in the Catskills, led by John Michelotti. Seeing it on a log was a really special moment, since my dad has been taking turkey tail since the beginning of his cancer treatment.

Turkey tail mushrooms are very thin, tough, and leathery in texture, so they aren't the most practical to use in cooking. You can, however, easily add powdered extracts of turkey tail into your cooking, add turkey tail tinctures to your smoothies, or make a tea with dried turkey tail mushrooms if you can get your hands on them.

Turkey tail's healing benefits:

- Immune system support
- Antitumor
- Antiviral
- Anti-inflammatory
- Can help fight infections
- Aids in digestion
- Adjunct to chemotherapy treatment

How to Get Started with Turkey Tail Mushrooms

- **A tincture, capsule, or powder extract.** As turkey tail is tough and leathery, it's usually taken medicinally as an extract (capsule, tincture, or powder). My dad has a bottle of turkey tail capsules on hand for traveling, and he consumes turkey tail powder or tincture extract in his daily smoothies. I take a turkey tail tincture as a preventative measure, or alongside my other daily medicinal immune support mushrooms (including chaga and reishi) when I feel like I might be coming down with something.

- **Add the powdered extract to food.** When my dad first got diagnosed and I was at home cooking for him a lot, I'd frequently add a spoonful of turkey tail extract powder into soups, stews, or other savory dishes. Find creative ways to sneak more turkey tail into your life!

- **Make turkey tail tea.** If you can find dried turkey tail mushrooms, you can make a tea with it just as you would any other mushroom. Add dried turkey tail mushrooms to a pot of boiling water and simmer for 1 hour. Add a squeeze of lemon and a teaspoon of honey, and sip.

Other medicinal mushrooms to look out for:

I've covered seven medicinal mushrooms in depth here in *The Rebel's Apothecary,* but there are many more varieties out there making magic happen in the world. A few other star mushrooms to look into are:

- *Agaricus blazei:* another potent cancer-fighting mushroom, often found in mushroom supplement blends

- Tremella: a moisturizing mushroom often used in skincare products

- Oyster: a common culinary mushroom that's very easy to grow at home! Cook it in any dish as you would with shiitake or maitake. Oyster mushrooms are antibacterial, can help lower cholesterol, and support the immune system—add it to your diet to support overall health.

Check the Resources section for some of my favorite mushroom books and websites to continue your mushroom adventure.

BUT WILL I GET HIGH? USING MEDICINAL MUSHROOMS WITHOUT FEAR

None of the mushrooms you've met so far in this book have any psychoactive or psychedelic effects at all. Rest assured that chaga, reishi, lion's mane, cordyceps, maitake, shiitake, and turkey tail are all safe and non-psychedelic. Of course, when you start experimenting with medicinal mushrooms, just like any plant or supplement, you'll want to take note of any effects you do notice and be aware of how you're feeling—but you won't get high from them.

MEDICINAL MUSHROOMS: A RECAP

- **Chaga:** immunity, detoxifying, anti-inflammatory
- **Reishi:** immunity, anti-stress, longevity
- **Lion's Mane:** brain health, mental focus, nerve support
- **Cordyceps:** energy, stamina, adrenal support
- **Maitake:** blood sugar stabilizing, immunity
- **Shiitake:** immunity, antiviral
- **Turkey Tail:** immunity, antiviral, antitumor

PART 2
EVERYDAY REBELS

Using Cannabis and Mushrooms for Daily Wellness

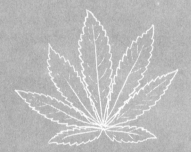

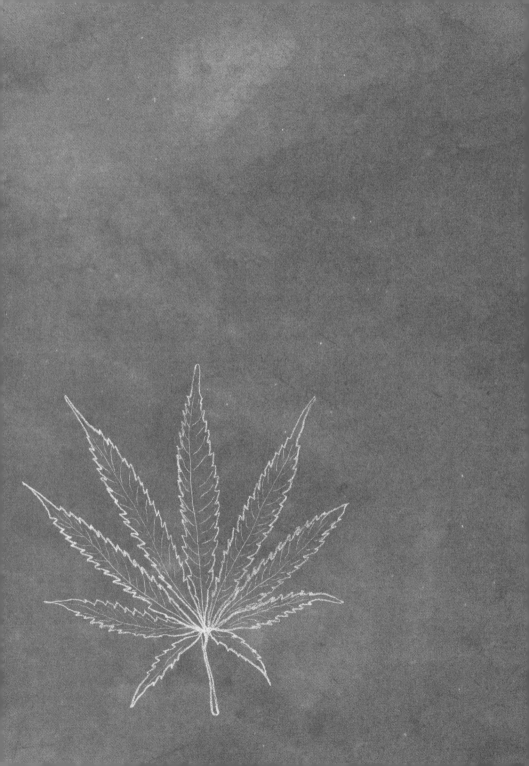

COOKING WITH CANNABIS
AND MEDICINAL MUSHROOMS

COOKING WITH CANNABIS

Before learning to cook with cannabis, the extent of my cannabis culinary skills included putting my CBD oil tincture into
my coffee or adding it to a batch of homemade cookies. That all
changed when I met Chef Chris Herko
of Seasoned Brooklyn, who frequently hosts cannabis-infused
dinner parties. I had never infused cannabis flower into food
before (the oldest trick in the
book when it comes to making cannabis edibles), so you can imagine
my fascination when he told me he
was a chef who makes cannabis-
infused meals.

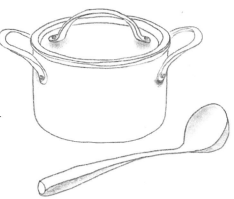

Chef Chris agreed to give me some cooking lessons using high-CBD strains of cannabis, and now I get to pass these CBD-infused delights on to you.

While you *can* simply add your CBD oil tincture directly into your food and drinks (it's a quick and easy way to infuse more cannabinoids into your everyday life), cooking with the cannabis flower is more of a culinary experience. Using CBD-rich strains of cannabis, you can create foundational ingredients like infused butter, coconut oil, and olive oil—and keep using them again and again to add healing cannabinoids to your favorite dishes.

During my cannabis cooking crash course, we infused all three of those foundational ingredients (butter, olive oil, and coconut oil), then cooked a full cannabis-infused meal so I could see firsthand exactly how to incorporate the infused butter and oil into different dishes.

We used infused olive oil for a salad dressing, infused butter on our salmon and veggies, and infused coconut oil to make sautéed peaches for dessert.

During the infused meal, we calculated that we consumed about 100 mg total of CBD each. That's a pretty high dose of CBD for most people—but because the strain we used had barely any THC in it, I didn't feel any intoxicating effects at all. I did, however, feel *very* relaxed, cheerful, and at ease about an hour after eating—and I slept very well that night. Thank you, CBD!

Now, I have CBD-infused butter, olive oil, and coconut oil in my kitchen ready to add to any dish, and I frequently buy CBD-rich cannabis flower to use in my cooking. These days, I make CBD cookies using my own homemade "cannabutter"—an incredibly delicious way to get your medicine!

Cannabis Cooking with High-CBD Strains

Historically, making cannabis edibles has been all about optimizing for THC content, for the strongest high. You may have had an experience with THC-rich edibles yourself—and if you took more than you meant to, you know very well that it's difficult to control dosing. The first time I ate a THC-rich edible was in college (at the MardiGrass cannabis festival in Nimbin, Australia), and I definitely wasn't expecting such strong effects—I had to lie down outside on a blanket for *hours!* When consuming edibles, it can be all too easy to ingest *way* too much THC, which converts to the more psychoactive 11-hydroxy-THC as it passes through the liver and digestive system.

Here in *The Rebel's Apothecary,* we are optimizing for high-CBD edibles, so we can get all the benefits of CBD while we enjoy our infused meal, without feeling intoxicated. While you can absolutely use any of the recipes in this book with high-THC cannabis if you so desire, my focus here is to use CBD-rich flower. Eating CBD-rich cannabis edibles may leave you feeling very relaxed, or even sleepy in some cases (CBD-infused dessert before bed, anyone?), and if you use the right kind of CBD flower to start with, you'll have a nonintoxicating, delicious experience infusing your medicine into everyday foods.

CBD Edibles as Medicine

Consuming CBD orally (i.e., eating it or drinking it) is often a less bioavailable way to consume it as a medicine (bioavailability refers to how much of the CBD is actually absorbed by the body), and it can be more difficult to control dosing. Everyone has a different digestive system, and dosing with edibles depends on how much CBD is contained in each serving, which can also be difficult to accurately measure. So, while it's definitely not the most streamlined method of consuming a specific dose of CBD, consuming an edible can be an easy and fun way to get more cannabinoids into your system and deliver some potent benefits.

Keep in mind that with edibles, you will likely need to wait longer to feel the effects than with other methods of delivery. It could be as long as 90–120 minutes until you feel any effects, rather than about 15 minutes with a tincture, or immediately with inhalation. While eating cannabis-infused food is definitely not the *fastest* way to symptom relief, the effects typically last a few hours longer. For this reason, many people swear by using edibles for pain and sleep, as the relaxing effects can last through the night.

So if you're looking to make a delicious dish, relax a little, get some extra cannabinoids into your body, and have some fun doing it . . . look no further than cooking with high-CBD cannabis!

First, Decide What You Want to Infuse

I love having a foundational, everyday-use CBD-infused product in my kitchen—olive oil, coconut oil, and butter are all great choices that you can keep on hand and use anytime you'd normally use butter or oil. Cannabis is fat soluble, or lipophilic (fat-loving), so consuming it in foods with fats will make the medicinal compounds more bioavailable.

Cannabutter is the ultimate cannabis-infused staple, especially for baked goods—so it can be a good place to start if you frequently use butter in your cooking. The best cooking fat to infuse is the one you love most and use most frequently. If you make salad dressings a lot, you may love an infused olive oil. If you're one who uses coconut oil for everything, make a batch of infused coconut oil to have on hand (which can also be fantastic on your skin as a topical).

Finding High-CBD Flower

If you've only had experience with CBD in the form of tinctures, capsules, or topicals, the day you decide to start infusing food with cannabis may be your first time handling raw CBD flower. It was for me. High-CBD flower is simply a cannabis strain that has been bred for high CBD levels and very low to negligible THC levels. It looks exactly like other cannabis flower you may have seen before, and usually people are surprised when I show it to them. "That's CBD? But it looks just like weed!" And it *is* weed—just not the kind that gets you high.

When you're making CBD-infused foods, you'll need to start with a high-CBD strain of raw cannabis—when I say "raw," I just mean it hasn't been heated (or decarboxylated) yet. You can find raw CBD flower at a dispensary, a CBD store, online (I've ordered from an Oregon-based company called Fields of Hemp), or perhaps from a friend who grew it in their backyard (you can order high-CBD seeds online, too)! No matter which way you choose to obtain them, make sure you're getting your hands on high-quality, lab-tested, CBD-rich buds. If you want to avoid feeling high, make sure you talk to your budtender and get a strain of cannabis with high percentages of CBD and low THC (either a hemp-based CBD strain with .3 percent or less THC, or a 30:1 CBD-to-THC strain if you have access to more options).

Again, the more THC in your raw flower, the greater the chance you'll get a visit from that extra-intoxicating surprise friend, 11-hydroxy-THC, after you eat.

Next: To Decarb or Not to Decarb?

As you may remember, raw cannabis flower needs to be decarboxylated ("decarbed," or heated) in order for THC and CBD to become activated. The natural compounds in the raw cannabis buds before heating are the acid cannabinoids, THCA and CBDA. When cannabis is heated, the A—or acid—molecule is dropped in the process, and the acid cannabinoids are converted to THC and CBD. If your cannabis isn't properly decarbed, you won't feel the effects of the THC or the CBD when you eat your edible.

Most often in cannabis-infused cooking, the goal is to activate as much THC or CBD as possible, but remember—the acid cannabinoids have their own health benefits, too.

When you're making a cannabis-infused cooking fat (such as a butter or an oil), you will be heating the butter or oil until it's liquid, adding the cannabis, and letting it simmer until the compounds in the cannabis are extracted from the plant and into the cooking liquid.

Although some decarboxylation will happen during this infusion process, some cannabis cooking enthusiasts swear by decarbing the raw flower in the oven *before* making an infused butter or oil. This way, they don't take the chance that it won't decarb fully in the heated liquid (which would result in a weaker infusion if you're optimizing for THC or CBD content).

Other cannabis cooks insist that the flower is, in fact, decarbed adequately during the infusion and subsequent meal-cooking process.

You can choose to decarb or not to decarb before you infuse, but I believe decarboxylation isn't necessary before infusing if you're not focused on the THC high. Since we're going for non-intoxicating infused foods here, we can afford to keep some of those friendly acid cannabinoids in there.

Raw cannabis is still medicinal, even when it hasn't been decarboxylated. Although the acid cannabinoids don't currently have as much popularity as THC and CBD, research has shown that both THCA and CBDA have anti-inflammatory, antinausea, and pain-relieving properties. This is why some people make juices or teas out of raw cannabis, to get the benefits of those acid cannabinoids without putting all the focus on THC or CBD.

As a bonus, you can even grind your raw cannabis and sprinkle it onto food as you would other herbs such as thyme or rosemary (as long as you like the taste of cannabis)!

If you're wondering about decarbing when it comes to CBD oil tinctures, all tinctures you purchase have already been decarbed (unless the tincture label specifically says "raw" and "CBDA" or "THCA" on it). When it comes to cooking with tinctures, as Chef Chris says: "It's as simple as putting whatever dosage you'd like into a drink, on top of food, or into any recipe."

How to Decarb Your Flower

Let's say you *do* want to fully decarb your flower before making an infusion, because the CBD or THC is what you care about most. Activating the CBD and THC in the raw cannabis without destroying cannabinoids and terpenes in the process is a matter of precision. The temperature at which cannabis begins to decarboxylate is about 220°F or 104°C. Many cannabis chefs recommend decarbing at temperatures between 220°F and 230°F, and not letting your cannabis heat to more than 300°F, as CBD can begin to evaporate at 320°F and terpenes begin to evaporate at temperatures above 300°F, too.

DECARB INSTRUCTIONS

Preheat your oven to 230°F. Break up your raw cannabis flower into small pieces with your hands (or grind the flower with a grinder) and spread the cannabis flower evenly on a rimmed baking sheet with parchment paper. The pieces of cannabis flower should be small enough that they can heat evenly all the way through. Bake for 30–45 minutes. It can be helpful to use an oven thermometer to make sure the temperature inside your oven is the same temperature it says on the outside, so you don't risk damaging your cannabinoids and terpenes at temperatures higher than 300°F. Keep an eye on your flower to make sure it doesn't burn. Once you've baked it and it's turned from green to a light brown color, you're decarbed and ready for cooking action.

HOW TO MAKE CBD-INFUSED BUTTER, OLIVE OIL, OR COCONUT OIL

Cannabutter or canna-oil is exactly what it sounds like—butter or oil, delightfully infused with cannabis. To make a cannabis-infused butter or oil, you have a couple of options. If you have cheesecloth, you can make a little sachet of cannabis flower and tie it up tightly, so no stray buds will get into your butter or oil. Alternatively, if you prefer a wilder way to cook it, you can just add the flower directly to the butter or oil—you'll have to strain it out afterward with a fine-mesh strainer.

Start with 8 oz. (1 cup) butter or oil and ¼ oz. of CBD-rich cannabis flower (adjust amounts as desired; calculations for determining how much CBD will be in your infusion are outlined in the next section).

If preferred, decarboxylate your flower before infusing.

Grind cannabis flower with an herb grinder (which you can find at a cannabis dispensary or smoke shop, or order online) or break buds into very tiny pieces with your hands and wrap in cheesecloth, tying it at the top to form a sachet.

Place the butter or oil in the top of a double boiler set over simmering water on low heat, so as not to burn it.

Add the sachet of CBD-rich cannabis flower to your butter or oil.

Simmer your sachet of cannabis in the butter or oil over low heat for about 2 hours. Both the butter and oil will turn green from the cannabis infusion, which is part of the fun. After 2 hours of simmering, you can remove the sachet or strain out the plant matter.

Use a kitchen thermometer to make sure the temperature of the butter or oil doesn't go above 300°F, so you can preserve the cannabinoids and terpenes.

Once it's infused, pour all of your beautiful green butter or oil into a separate container and squeeze or press the sachet (watch out, it's hot!) until all the butter or oil has been removed. If you didn't use a sachet and you just simmered the nuggets of cannabis right in the liquid, just get a very fine mesh strainer, strain out the plant matter, and discard it. Use the butter or oil as you normally would with any food.

How to Calculate the Amount of CBD in Your Butter or Oil

In order to calculate the amount of CBD that will be infused into your butter or oil, you must know two things: how much flower you have (in grams) and the percentage of CBD in that flower (all dispensaries will have this information available when you purchase the flower).

Let's say you have 1 g of CBD-rich cannabis flower that measures in at 15 percent CBD.

BECAUSE 1 G EQUALS 1000 MG, THERE ARE
150 MG TOTAL CBD IN YOUR 1 G OF DRY HERB
(15 PERCENT OF 1000 MG = 150 MG).

Weight conversions, for reference (this is the dry weight of the flower, not the amount of CBD):

¼ OZ. OF FLOWER = 7 G

⅛ OZ. OF FLOWER = 3.5 G

Now that we understand that calculation, let's pretend we're cooking with ¼ oz. of cannabis flower, or 7 g. Since we know there's 150 mg of CBD per gram, the total amount of CBD we have available is 1050 mg.

This calculation is the total amount of CBD available once it has been decarboxylated. If you choose not to decarboxylate your cannabis flower first, you will have varying amounts of CBD and CBDA present.

Keep in mind, however, that this is the maximum number of milligrams of CBD that could potentially be consumed. It will likely be less, due to a few different factors: All the CBD may not be extracted from the flower into the butter or oil, and you will not absorb all of the CBD through the digestive tract. So while it's helpful to understand ballpark ranges for edibles, remember that consuming cannabis edibles is not the most accurate way to get a very specific dose.

Calculating the Amount of CBD in 1 Tablespoon of Butter or Oil

¼ OZ. (OR 7 G) OF CANNABIS FLOWER, DECARBOXYLATED

15 PERCENT CBD

150 MG CBD PER GRAM, 1050 MG MAXIMUM TOTAL
AVAILABLE CBD

8 OZ. BUTTER OR OIL = 16 TBSP.

THIS EQUALS ABOUT 65.6 MG TOTAL CBD PER TABLESPOON,
IF EVENLY DISTRIBUTED THROUGHOUT THE BUTTER OR OIL.
(1050 MG OF CBD DIVIDED BY 16 TBSP. OF BUTTER).

Let's say we're using 4 Tbsp. (¼ cup) of cannabutter in a batch of cookies. In this scenario, we'd have about 260 mg of CBD spread throughout the entire batch of cookies.

260 MG / 12 COOKIES = ABOUT 22 MG TOTAL CBD PER COOKIE.
ADJUST AMOUNTS AS DESIRED.

General Cannabis Cooking Tips:

- Whenever consuming cannabis edibles, expect to wait at least 60–90 minutes to feel the effects.

- Cannabis compounds are fat-soluble, so they need to be infused in a fat (which is why we use butter, olive oil, or coconut oil).

- Whether you're adding a CBD tincture to your food or infusing oil or butter with CBD flower, make sure to spread the CBD as evenly as possible throughout the meal, for equal dosing in each serving.

- To make infused honey, add CBD oil tincture or infused coconut oil to honey and blend.

- Most canna-chefs aim to stay below 300°F when doing infusions.

- Use lab-tested cannabis to ensure the math on recipes is as correct as possible.

- Triple-check your math—especially if you're using any THC in your recipes.

- In any soup, stew, or broth you're making in a pot, you can add a sachet of CBD-rich cannabis flower to infuse cannabinoids into your meal! Remember to remove the sachet before serving.

- If you like the taste of cannabis, you can sprinkle either raw or decarboxylated ground cannabis into your dishes, as you would any with other herb.

- If you want to infuse butter and oil regularly, you may want to look into the Magical Butter machine—it's a countertop infuser that will infuse any herb into butter or oil easily.

- If you're consuming edibles that contain any amount of THC, go very slowly. It's easy to overdo it, and you can always eat more later.

Using Cannabis-Infused Butter or Oil

When using your cannabis-infused butter or oil for cooking, the lower the temperature, the better if you want to preserve the most medicine. If you cook your cannabis oil or butter at high temperatures (i.e., sautéing) or put it over direct high heat, some of the cannabinoids and terpenes can be destroyed. This doesn't mean you can't do it—plenty of cannabis chefs use their cannabutter to scramble eggs or make stir-fry with canna–coconut oil—but if you're going to sauté in a pan, do so over low heat. Baking isn't a threat to the cannabinoids and terpenes—the internal temperature of baked goods doesn't go above 300°F, even if you're baking at temperatures higher than that.

Ideas for using your infused cannabutter or canna-oil:

- Use the olive oil in salad dressings

- Add the coconut oil to any smoothie

- Drizzle the olive oil on top of soups or stews

- Make CBD guacamole with a swirl of the olive oil

- Make a Bulletproof-style cannabis coffee by blending infused coconut oil or butter into your coffee

- Add cannabutter or canna–coconut oil to any baked dessert or baked dish

- Add the infused olive oil to hummus or dips

- Spread cannabutter on your favorite sourdough bread

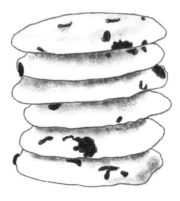

GLUTEN-FREE CBD CHOCOLATE-CHIP (OR BLUEBERRY) COOKIES

This is a CBD-rich twist on one of the most popular cookie recipes on my blog, and my new favorite way to use cannabutter. I make these cookies for every holiday, and often give them to people I love as gifts. I've upgraded my normal recipe to include cannabutter (you can also use canna–coconut oil here instead of butter) to infuse these cookies with CBD. An alternative to this recipe that I love making in the summertime is blueberry cookies—I swap the chocolate for fresh blueberries, using the same recipe.

Makes 12 cookies

2 cups almond flour

½ tsp. baking soda

¼ tsp. sea salt

¼ cup honey

1 Tbsp. vanilla extract

¼ cup CBD-infused coconut oil *or* grass-fed butter (page 140)—
if you don't have infused butter or oil, you can use plain butter
or coconut oil, and add a few dropperfuls of your favorite CBD
tincture, at your preferred dosage. Keep in mind, a flavored tincture
will affect the taste.

1 (2-oz.) bar of high-quality dark chocolate—I use Hu Kitchen
chocolate bars. You can substitute ½ cup of fresh blueberries here
to make the blueberry version of these cookies.

Preheat oven to 350°F.

Add almond flour, baking soda, and sea salt to food processor or high-speed blender and mix well. (You can simply stir with a fork or whisk instead of blending/food-processing, but the texture of the dough won't be as smooth.)

Add honey, vanilla, and coconut oil or butter to the mixture.

Mix well (or pulse if you're using a food processor) until it becomes a dough.

Transfer dough to a bowl.

Chop up chocolate bar and add the chocolate pieces to the dough.

Roll dough into 1-inch balls (using 1–2 Tbsp. dough for each cookie) and line on cookie sheet on parchment paper. Pat down with fingers. If using blueberries, add 2–3 blueberries to each cookie once the balls of dough are on the cookie sheet and press blueberries into the dough.

Bake for 6–9 minutes (yes, that's it!), until golden brown. Let cool before serving.

SAUTÉED PEACHES AND FIGS WITH CANNA-COCONUT OIL

CONTRIBUTED BY CHEF CHRIS HERKO

Chef Chris made this for dessert during my cannabis cooking lesson, and the flavors were amazing. I love fruit for dessert, especially with a savory bit of ricotta and a pinch of sea salt. You can use your infused cannabutter or canna-oil here. Remember, it's best to use cannabis cooking fats at lower temperatures, so keep it as low as possible to preserve the most cannabinoids and terpenes.

4 servings

2 peaches

1 pint fresh figs

1 Tbsp. infused coconut oil *or* infused butter (page 140)

1 Tbsp. honey

1 cup ricotta

Maldon Sea Salt

½ cup pepitas, toasted

3 sprigs thyme

Zest of 1 lime

Remove pits from the peaches and cut into slices. Cut all figs in half lengthwise.

Melt infused coconut oil or butter in a pan over low heat and add figs and peaches. Cook on low until tender, 3–5 minutes. Let sit in warm pan until ready to plate.

While the fruit is cooking, mix honey and ricotta in a bowl—add a pinch of salt if desired.

Smear a scoop of the ricotta/honey mixture onto each plate and scoop equal portions of fruit over top of the ricotta. Sprinkle with toasted pepitas.

Remove thyme sprigs from stems and sprinkle on top as a garnish.

Sprinkle with lime zest and top with a pinch of Maldon Sea Salt.

INFUSED ORANGE VINAIGRETTE

CONTRIBUTED BY CHEF CHRIS HERKO

This is just one of many ways you can use CBD-infused olive oil! Use this bright, citrusy CBD-infused dressing on your favorite salad. If you don't have CBD-infused olive oil, you can add your favorite unflavored CBD tincture to this recipe at your preferred dose. This dressing is wonderful on a salad of mixed greens with chopped beets and feta.

Makes 2 cups of dressing

4 Tbsp. balsamic vinegar

1 shallot, coarsely chopped

1 clove garlic, coarsely chopped

½ cup orange juice (fresh-squeezed if possible; from about 2 large oranges)

Zest of 2 oranges (optional)

½ tsp. salt

½ tsp. black pepper

1 tsp. Dijon mustard

½ cup CBD-infused extra-virgin olive oil (page 140)

Add all ingredients to a blender except oil.

Blend until smooth.

While blending, slowly drizzle oil into blender in a thin stream, to emulsify.

Serve or keep refrigerated. Keeps for 1 month.

Shake well (as oil will separate) to re-emulsify before using.

CBD TAHINI DRESSING
("POUR THIS ON EVERYTHING" SAUCE)

Tahini dressing is my all-time favorite sauce to pour on my salads and roasted veggies. I always use olive oil when making it, and using CBD-infused olive oil makes this dressing even more nourishing and delicious. My suggestion is to make a pan of roasted veggies (brussels sprouts, sweet potatoes, and broccoli are all great choices), and drizzle this tahini sauce all over them. And while you're at it, pour it on any other savory dish you can think of! Another favorite way to use it is on top of a fresh arugula salad with sliced cucumbers.

Makes about 1 cup of dressing—double or triple the recipe and keep it in a jar in the fridge if you love it as much as I do! Generally, equal parts water and tahini work well—but feel free to add either more water (thinner dressing) or more tahini (thicker dressing).

½ cup tahini (sesame seed paste)

½ cup water

2 Tbsp. CBD-infused olive oil (page 140), or 2 Tbsp. olive oil + your preferred dosage of your CBD tincture, preferably unflavored

1 clove garlic

¼ cup lemon juice (juice of 1 lemon), plus more to taste

½ tsp. sea salt, plus more to taste

½ tsp. black pepper

Add all ingredients to a blender and blend.

Add more water or olive oil to make a thinner sauce, and add more tahini for a thicker sauce.

Add more salt or lemon juice to taste.

Once well blended, pour over salads, veggies, or any savory dish! You can also use this tahini sauce as a dip for raw veggies.

You'll find more CBD-infused recipes sprinkled throughout the rest of this book.

COOKING WITH MEDICINAL MUSHROOMS

Of all the mushrooms we're focusing on in *The Rebel's Apothecary*, there are three we've learned about so far that are considered "culinary," and therefore great for cooking—shiitake, maitake, and lion's mane. Cooking with mushrooms is one of the easiest ways to infuse their healing properties into your life.

Because of their texture, taste, and consistency, reishi, chaga, turkey tail, and cordyceps are all typically extracted for use in teas, powders, tinctures, or capsules rather than cooked and eaten. You can, however, add the powdered extracts of these mushrooms into any dish to enhance the medicinal properties of your food.

There are other incredible culinary mushrooms you might see at your local grocery store, and they have plenty of nutritional properties, too—so have fun experimenting with mushrooms like chanterelles, oysters, or trumpets.

If you want to try your hand at mushroom cooking (and I suggest you do), you can't go wrong by cooking any edible mushroom in a pan with butter, garlic, salt, and pepper. If you don't eat dairy, you can use coconut oil instead of butter, which adds a delicious coconut flavor to the mushrooms.

To prepare them, slice or chop up your mushrooms, put them into a pan with butter or oil, a chopped-up clove of garlic, and salt and pepper to taste. Cook them until they're browned and have a slight crisp to them.

The cooking time will be different with each mushroom and will also depend on how much water is in the mushroom—if you wash them before cooking, you will want to dry them well first to let the water soak out. Otherwise, you'll lengthen your cooking time because the water will have to cook out before they can get crispy.

Shiitakes are easy to find and very versatile, so you can throw them into the pan anytime you're cooking veggies. Maitake mushrooms, like shiitakes, are perfect when sautéed or baked. If I'm making a salad, eggs, rice dish, or pasta dish, I love to sauté either shiitakes or maitakes in a pan separately, and add them into the dish once they're crisp.

If you're cooking lion's mane mushrooms, it's often suggested not to wash them first if you can get away with it (unless there's a lot of dirt on them, of course). If you can brush the dirt off easily without washing, do so. Those babies soak up water like a sponge! When cooking with lion's mane, slice or chop the lion's mane and cook in a pan with butter or coconut oil until golden brown, and sprinkle with sea salt.

Cooking with Dried Mushrooms

Dried mushrooms can add a lot of flavor to any dish. In order to cook with them, you'll want to soak them first to rehydrate them. Add your dried mushrooms to a bowl of warm water and let them soak for 20 minutes. After 20 minutes, you can remove the mushrooms, rinse, and add them to sauces, stews, stir-fries, eggs, rice dishes, or any other dish where you want to pack in some mushroom flavor. You can also use the soaking water, but strain it with a fine-mesh strainer first to get rid of any "grit" from the mushrooms that has settled at the bottom of the bowl.

The only time you don't need to rehydrate your mushrooms is if you're making tea or broth (two recipes are coming up next!)—in those cases, you'll just add the dried mushrooms to water.

You'll find medicinal mushroom recipes sprinkled throughout the rest of this book—some from me, some from friends and chefs. Next up are a few recipes using the edible cooking mushrooms—shiitake, maitake, and lion's mane. Get creative with your mushroom cooking, and enjoy the health-enhancing benefits!

SHIITAKE OR MAITAKE BACON

Mushroom bacon has become one of my medicinal mushroom staple foods, and one of my favorite things to make for dinner with my friends. Mushroom bacon adds a satisfying (and medicinal) crunch to any salad or meal. I've tried this recipe with shiitake and maitake mushrooms, and it works well with both. Don't blame me if you get addicted to eating mushrooms this way!

> About 2 cups chopped shiitake (stems removed) or maitake mushrooms, cut into thin slices—enough to line a baking sheet.
>
> 1 Tbsp. coconut oil
>
> 1 Tbsp. tamari (wheat-free soy sauce), or coconut aminos if you're soy-free

Preheat oven to 375°F.

Add the sliced mushrooms to a bowl and gently coat them with the coconut oil.

Line a rimmed baking sheet with parchment paper, and arrange the mushrooms on the parchment paper so they aren't overlapping one another.

Bake mushrooms for 30 minutes, or until they are lightly browned and crispy. During the last 5 minutes of cooking, remove pan from oven, sprinkle tamari or coconut aminos over the mushrooms, and put back into the oven. (The reason to wait until the end of cooking is because the tamari can burn easily if you add it at the beginning.)

Remove mushrooms from the pan and put them on a paper towel to blot the oil if needed, just as you would regular bacon. Add to any meal, or eat them alone as a snack!

Note: Just as with regular bacon, you can also make your mushroom bacon in a pan—use the same recipe but put the chopped-up mushrooms in a skillet instead of in the oven. Cook with coconut oil, and splash with tamari or aminos right before removing from the heat. Transfer the mushroom bacon to a paper towel to blot out oil before serving.

MY FAVORITE MASSAGED KALE SALAD (GREAT FOR MUSHROOM BACON!):

Makes 2 servings

1 bunch of raw kale, chopped

Juice of 1 lemon

1 avocado, skin and pit removed

Pinch of sea salt

½ cup cherry tomatoes, cut in half

½ cup feta, crumbled

½ cup mushroom bacon (page 154)

Add kale pieces to bowl and squeeze lemon juice over the kale. Add the avocado and pinch of sea salt to the bowl.

Massage the lemon, avocado, and salt into the kale with your hands until the kale is soft (about 5 minutes). Add the cherry tomatoes, feta, and the mushroom bacon. Mix gently and enjoy!

LION'S MANE BRAISED IN COCONUT

CONTRIBUTED BY CHEF SEAMUS MULLEN

This recipe is from my friend Seamus Mullen, an award-winning New York City chef, restaurateur, and cookbook author. His meals are always both delicious and health focused, and in this recipe he takes lion's mane cooking to the next level. Lion's mane has the texture of lobster or crab, and it pairs perfectly with the coconut milk, lime, and cilantro here. The flavors in this dish are out of this world!

Makes 2 servings

2 Tbsp. coconut oil

4 cups fresh lion's mane mushrooms, chopped

½ cup unsweetened coconut milk

2 cloves garlic, thinly sliced

Salt and pepper, to taste

Zest and juice of 1 lime

Fresh cilantro, as garnish

Heat coconut oil in a sauté pan over high heat, add chopped lion's mane to the pan, and quickly brown lion's mane.

When lion's mane is golden brown, add coconut milk and sliced garlic. Bring to a boil, then reduce to a simmer for 5 minutes.

After 5 minutes, remove from heat.

Season with salt and pepper and finish with lime zest, lime juice, and fresh cilantro to taste.

SHIITAKE MUSHROOM BROTH

CONTRIBUTED BY CHEF MARCO CANORA

Chef Marco Canora's Hearth Restaurant is my favorite restaurant in all of Manhattan. He also owns Brodo Bone Broth Company—they make the best bone broths and mushroom broths in the city. He's contributed this savory shiitake broth using dried shiitakes, which is perfect for boosting immunity during those cold winter months (or anytime!).

Makes about 4 quarts of broth—you can cut this recipe in half to make less, or double it to make more. Put the extra broth in the freezer and use it in soups or stews or as a sipping broth anytime.

2 large onions, peeled

1 tsp. extra-virgin olive oil

2 cups dried shiitake mushrooms

6 celery stalks, coarsely chopped

2 bay leaves

¼ bunch fresh thyme

½ Tbsp. black peppercorns

1 whole head of garlic, cut in half

Fine sea salt to taste

Cut 1 onion in half crosswise. Coarsely chop the remaining onion and set aside.

Heat olive oil in a skillet and add the halved onion, cut-side down. Brown the onion halves for 4–5 minutes without moving them.

Place the browned onions and the rest of the ingredients (except salt) in an 8-qt. pot (or a 16-qt. pot if doubling the recipe). Add cold water to cover all ingredients by 2 or 3 inches.

Bring to boil over high heat for about 40 minutes, skimming any foam every 15–20 minutes.

Reduce heat to low and simmer for 2–3 hours, skimming occasionally.

Strain the broth through a fine mesh strainer. Remove and discard all solid ingredients.

Season with salt to taste.

Keeps for 5 days in the refrigerator and 6 months in the freezer.

SHIITAKE GRAVY

This is the best gravy I've ever tasted in my life. It's thick, creamy, savory, and everything you could want in a gravy. As an added bonus, it's gluten-free, dairy free, and full of potent shiitake medicine! I make this gravy at every holiday dinner, and it's everyone's favorite part of the meal. Throughout the years, I've had many of my blog readers start making this gravy at their own holiday dinners, with much fanfare. Even the people in your life who don't think they like mushrooms will be instantly converted with this gravy!

Makes 3–4 cups of gravy, depending on how much water you add

6 Tbsp. extra-virgin olive oil

2 cups chopped and stemmed shiitake mushrooms

1 cup chopped yellow onion

2 cloves garlic, chopped

½ cup brown rice flour (or other gluten-free flour)

2 cups water

¼ cup wheat-free tamari

2 tsp. fresh thyme, stripped from stem

2 tsp. fresh rosemary, stripped from stem

1 tsp. freshly ground black pepper

Add 3 Tbsp. olive oil to a sauté pan over medium heat. Add mushrooms, onions, and garlic. Cook until onions are translucent and mushrooms are soft (about 5 minutes).

In a separate pan, add brown rice flour, and whisk in the remaining 3 Tbsp. oil, water, tamari, herbs, and black pepper. Bring to a boil and whisk until gravy is thick (about 10 minutes).

Add the gravy mix and onion/mushroom/garlic mix to a blender and blend until smooth. If your gravy is too thick, add more water a little bit at a time until you reach your desired consistency. Make sure to hold your hand over the top of the blender with a towel while blending, so the hot gravy doesn't pop the top off!

Pour hot gravy over all of your favorite holiday foods.

GRILLED MAITAKE MUSHROOMS

CONTRIBUTED BY CHEF WILL HICKOX

Here's a simple and delicious way to cook maitake mushrooms, from my friend Chef Will Hickox. Chef Will's master cooking skills have graced the kitchens of some of the best New York City restaurants, and here he teaches us to make maitake on the grill—an awesome idea for outdoor BBQs. If you don't have a grill, you can easily make this recipe in a pan on your stove using the same directions.

Makes 2–4 servings, depending on size of mushroom

1 clove garlic, peeled

1-inch piece of fresh ginger, peeled

3 Tbsp. extra-virgin olive oil

1 maitake head, sliced in quarters

Zest and juice of ½ lemon

2 Tbsp. finely minced parsley

Sea salt, to taste

Heat up grill, on low heat.

In a bowl, grate garlic and ginger with a Microplane into olive oil.

Toss maitake with half of the oil mixture, plus sea salt to taste.

Grill maitake until soft and slightly charred, turning as needed to prevent burning. Remove from grill.

Add lemon zest to the remaining half of the oil mixture, and add minced parsley.

Add lemon juice to oil mixture.

Dress the grilled maitake with the oil/lemon juice/parsley mixture.

Enjoy!

MAITAKE MINT TEA

CONTRIBUTED BY TRADD COTTER

This is the tea that was always on tap at Mushroom Mountain in South Carolina, where I attended a medicinal mushroom seminar. Tradd Cotter is the author of *Organic Mushroom Farming and Mycordemediation* and grows an abundance of different medicinal mushrooms at his research facility. This maitake tea is easy to make, and another great way to get the immune-enhancing, blood-sugar-stabilizing effects of the dancing mushroom.

Makes 2 servings

4 cups water

2 Tbsp. dried maitake pieces

10 fresh mint leaves

A touch of honey, to taste (optional)

In a pot, bring water to a boil and then reduce to a low simmer. Add dried maitake and fresh mint leaves and simmer for 15 minutes. Pour liquid through strainer into a mug, and sip. If you'd like to add sweetener, add a touch of honey.

REBEL'S GREEN SMOOTHIE

Green smoothies have been one of my favorite go-to healthy recipes for over a decade now—I've been making them ever since I first started my health coach training at the Institute for Integrative Nutrition. I love a creamy, cinnamon-packed green smoothie—I use a little bit of avocado to get that creaminess. Here, I've upgraded one of my all-time favorite green smoothie recipes to "rebel style," adding both CBD and mushrooms!

Makes 1 serving

1 cup coconut water

1 cup spinach

1–2 Tbsp. almond butter

¼ avocado

1 tsp. cinnamon (or more to taste)

½ tsp. vanilla extract

1 tsp. mushroom powder extract (a mushroom blend, or a single mushroom—your choice!)

1 dropperful of CBD oil at your preferred dosage (a mint chocolate flavor is amazing here, but unflavored works well, too)

Pinch of sea salt

Add all ingredients to a blender, blend, and sip. Coconut water makes this smoothie slightly sweet, but if you want even more sweetness, you can use ½ banana instead of avocado, or add a few drops of vanilla stevia.

MAKE YOUR OWN MUSHROOM TINCTURE

DIRECTIONS PROVIDED BY JOHN MICHELOTTI
OF CATSKILL FUNGI

If you're the DIY type, you'll love creating your own medicinal mushroom tincture at home. At a workshop in Brooklyn, I learned to make a chaga tincture under the guidance of John Michelotti of Catskill Fungi. He was kind enough to share his chaga tincture recipe with us here—and he says we can use this to make tinctures with any of the medicinal mushrooms in this book! At Catskill Fungi, the tinctures are all triple-extracted (in alcohol, cold water, and hot water). This ensures you get all the medicine from the mushrooms—including beta glucans (hot water), triterpenes (alcohol), and enzymes/metabolites (cold water), all of which have health benefits. Happy tincture making!

STEP 1: ALCOHOL EXTRACT

1 tsp. powdered chaga

2 fl oz. (¼ cup) high-proof alcohol—93 percent alcohol or 186 proof

Add both to a tincture bottle, keep on your countertop, and shake every day for 4 weeks.

After 4 weeks, strain the mushroom from the liquid and set liquid aside. We will be using the strained mushroom material in the next step.

STEP 2: COLD-WATER EXTRACT

Take the mushroom powder that was strained from alcohol and add it to 2 fl oz. (¼ cup) pure cold water.

Keep refrigerated and shake every 8 hours for 24 hours.

After 24 hours, strain mushroom from liquid, keep the liquid, and store in fridge. We will use the strained mushroom material in the next step.

STEP 3: HOT-WATER EXTRACT

Take the mushroom that was strained from the alcohol and cold water, and place in a pot. Add 6 fl oz. (¾ cup) water, heat to boiling on the stove below 180°F (the stove's low setting) until it's reduced to 2 fl oz (¼ cup).

Strain mushroom from liquid, discard mushroom, and let liquid cool.

STEP 4: COMBINE ALL 3 LIQUIDS

Combine 2 oz. liquid from each extraction into a 6-oz. tincture bottle. Store out of direct sunlight.

Take 2 dropperfuls per day. Makes a 3-month supply of triple-extracted chaga extract.

This process can be done with any of the other medicinal mushrooms as well.

CANNABIS AND MUSHROOM WELLNESS PROTOCOLS

Now that you're familiar with the many healing benefits that cannabis and medicinal mushrooms can provide, it's time to learn how to use them for some of the most everyday common wellness concerns. As a health coach, I talk to people about wellness constantly. Some of the most common things I hear people struggling with are sleep, pain, anxiety, stress, energy, focus, mood, and immunity.

I've provided cannabis and mushroom suggestions to help with all of these concerns in the following sections (and added tips for skincare and sex drive, too!). As always, keep in mind that your body and health situation are unique, and you will likely need to experiment a little bit to find the relief you're looking for. And if I haven't said it enough already, work with a doctor or other health care professional to find what works best for you.

Let's discover exactly how cannabis and mushrooms can support you in getting better sleep, having more energy, enhancing your mood, and generally feeling healthier and more vibrant every day.

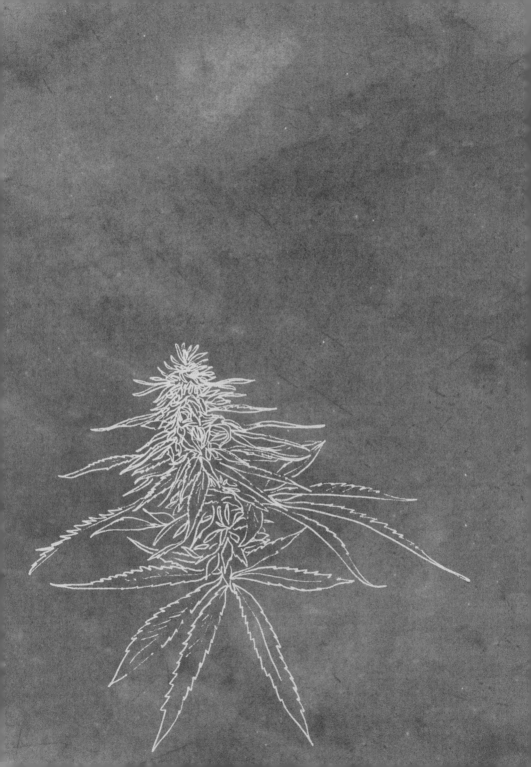

DEEPEN YOUR SLEEP

We all know the despair and exhaustion that comes with having a sleepless night—or, worse, many sleepless nights in a row. If you've experienced sleep deprivation or insomnia, you know—the next day, everything in life just feels *so* much harder to navigate. It feels impossible to concentrate, decision making is difficult, and even the smallest things can feel completely overwhelming. Your throat might start to get scratchy, and your immune system starts to feel weaker.

Lack of sleep can affect every aspect of our well-being. It can lead to higher levels of depression and anxiety, and the less we sleep, the more our mental capacity is diminished. In addition, sleep deprivation can cause us to gain weight or to keep unwanted weight on.

OUR BODIES NEED SLEEP TO REGENERATE AND HEAL.

Life without sleep is unmanageable, and while we know getting a good night's sleep is the only thing that will truly help, our anxiety about not sleeping can keep us up yet *another* night. Going without sleep can be a miserable cycle, so finding relief from insomnia is one of the greatest gifts.

Dr. Dustin Sulak says that in his practice, tackling insomnia or sleep problems is usually the first thing he focuses on, since many other issues clear themselves up after sleep gets back on track.

"Correcting disturbed sleep may be the highest-impact thing you can do for your health," he says.

So how can we sleep longer and deeper, naturally?

Managing stress and maintaining a higher level of overall health can be major contributors to a better sleep experience, and cannabis and mushrooms are both primed to be some of our greatest sleep helpers.

Here's how cannabis and medicinal mushrooms could turn out to be key players in your healthy sleep routine, along with a few other sleep tricks I'll share with you.

CBD AND SLEEP

When I first tried CBD, I'd been struggling with sleep for a few years. My body felt like it was on high alert all the time, and I had an anxious energy running through me during the night. Even if my mind was relaxed and I wasn't feeling stressed out about anything in particular, my body still had a hard time relaxing. All I wanted was to be able to drift into sleep and stay asleep for the whole night, but this kind of slumber usually evaded me.

I remember exactly the way I felt the first time I took CBD oil at night. I had ordered a full-spectrum CBD oil from a company called SupHERBals, recommended by a friend, and I was excited to try it. I bought it in tincture form, because my research had taught me that a tincture can work more quickly than a capsule for anxiety. Since I believed it was anxiety that was keeping me from falling asleep, this seemed promising.

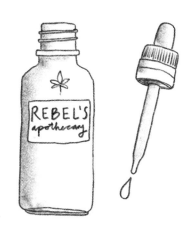

I took about half a dropperful, which was about 15 milligrams of CBD. I wasn't expecting any kind of miracle, but I kid you not—that night, my body was actually able to relax into a deep sleep. I woke up the next morning, knowing I'd had a full night's sleep, and I couldn't believe it. It had been so long since my body was able to fully rest without being on high alert all night. I was sold.

The difference that the CBD made for me felt physical—the CBD oil calmed my nervous system enough that I wasn't jumpy, agitated, and on edge. It wasn't that the CBD felt like a sedative—it just seemed to help calm that agitation in my nervous system. It stopped me from feeling anxious and allowed me to take a deep exhale.

CBD itself isn't a sleep promoter, necessarily—meaning it's not a sedative. Some people find it helpful for sleep, but others find it to be stimulating or wake-promoting. If someone finds relief from insomnia from CBD, it is likely a result of the CBD calming their anxiety or relieving their pain—the issue that was originally keeping them awake in the first place. If your reason for not being able to sleep is something like stress, anxiety, or pain, CBD could calm you down enough, or reduce your pain, so you're able to relax into sleep.

I consider CBD to be one of the most important parts of my sleep regimen today, because of the way it soothes my anxiety. I have a few other sleep helpers, too, and they all contribute to my personal sleep entourage. I take magnesium, wear a sleep mask, and turn on a sound machine for white noise. But CBD gives my nervous system exactly what it needs to chill out enough to drift off into dreamland.

According to Project CBD, the endocannabinoid system is involved in regulating sleep cycles—our ability to be awake, fall asleep, stay asleep, and wake up feeling rested. We have cannabinoid receptors all throughout our central nervous system, including the parts of the brain that regulate our sleep-wake cycles, so it makes sense that cannabis would have an impact on sleep. As we've learned, CBD can lead to higher levels of that "bliss molecule," anandamide, and interestingly, it turns out that anandamide can be found in the brain at higher levels at night, helping to generate deeper sleep.

CBD taken with THC has been shown—for some people—to be more effective for sleep than CBD on its own. Many people report that consuming THC (particularly in the form of edibles or capsules, which can be longer-lasting) help with achieving a deeper night's sleep. Keep in mind, however, that high amounts of THC are associated with sleep disruption. This is where that "therapeutic window" comes into play—you will likely have to experiment a bit to find what your body responds to best.

Best methods of delivery for CBD and sleep:

- Tincture under the tongue, 15 minutes before bedtime
- Capsule, swallowed, 30 minutes before bedtime
- Edible, eaten or in a drink, 60 minutes before bedtime
- Topical, applied to the body, to reduce pain that could be causing sleeplessness, immediately before bedtime
- Inhalation, immediately before bedtime

Because tinctures work more quickly than capsules or edibles do, a tincture can be better at helping you fall asleep, while a capsule or edible could be better for keeping you asleep longer. If you really want to double down, you could take a tincture *and* a capsule or edible before bed—that way, you take care of the falling asleep *and* the staying asleep. Be mindful of THC content if you choose to do this, as too much THC may disrupt your sleep (and can inhibit dreaming!).

When it comes to dosing for sleep, start slow. The goal is to find that sweet spot—how much do you need to relax into a blissful sleep?

USING A HIGH-THC PRODUCT FOR SLEEP, WITHOUT THE HIGH

A topical massage oil with both CBD and THC can be extremely relaxing for your body, while relieving your pain at the same time. Massage the oil into your skin (or have your partner give you a relaxing massage with a cannabis-infused body oil) for extra full-body relaxation prior to sleep. As it's rare to feel any intoxicating effects from a topical, you won't get high from the THC—but your body will feel relaxed and soothed. After all, your skin has an abundance of cannabinoid receptors. On nights when I'm having a particularly difficult time falling asleep or I'm feeling activated or energized at bedtime, I'll take a dose of full-spectrum CBD oil in tincture form, and then I'll slowly massage a CBD/THC oil into my skin. It's incredibly relaxing, especially after a hot shower or bath. I found the CBD/THC massage oil at a dispensary—so if you don't have access to THC products where you live, a CBD massage oil will work just fine.

If it's pain that's keeping you awake, it may be helpful to try a topical or transdermal cream, balm, or roll-on (with both CBD and THC in it, if you can find it) that you apply locally to wherever it hurts. CBD and THC together can be extremely pain-relieving, and topicals can be a great way to relieve pain that keeps you up at night.

One of my favorite products for pain is a 1:1 CBD-to-THC "transdermal compound," which you can likely find at a dispensary (my favorite is from Mary's Medicinals). I broke my tailbone a few years ago, and I still experience intermittent pain from it, which can disrupt my sleep. This transdermal compound also helps tremendously with menstrual cramps that can keep me awake. These days, with my cannabinoid pain arsenal, I'm usually able to melt easily into rest.

Cannabis varieties with higher amounts of the terpenes myrcene and linalool, and the cannabinoid CBN (which is a breakdown product of THC when it gets older), are thought to be more relaxing and sedating. If you're at a dispensary looking for a more sleepy cannabis variety to help you rest, you'll want to check that lab test for myrcene, linalool, and CBN, or ask the budtenders to direct you to strains that have terpene and cannabinoid profiles that typically produce an "indica" effect.

If you have a CBD or THC tincture and want to make your own massage oil, you can add a dropperful of your CBD tincture to a spoonful of coconut oil, sesame oil, or almond oil as a carrier (or your favorite lotion) and massage it into your skin.

MUSHROOMS AND SLEEP

If you want a medicinal mushroom that will help you relax into the evening, look no further than queen reishi. Reishi mushrooms have a calming effect on the nervous system, which makes reishi tea a perfect wind-down drink. If you've had a long day, a cup of reishi tea (or a reishi tincture) will be your new favorite nightcap. As with CBD, reishi is not a sedative, but it can be very calming to the nervous system.

Reishi tea is also a really wonderful alternative to winding down with a glass of wine or other alcoholic beverage. In fact, alcohol can disrupt your sleep, preventing you from truly getting that deep rest you crave. If you're used to relying on alcohol to help you fall asleep, in the long run you'll likely end up feeling more sleep deprived.

Reishi, however, can help to activate the body's natural sleep cycles, which can help coax you into a healthier sleep rhythm.

"Reishi is so gentle—you can take it at night within an hour of bed to help promote sleep. It's calming for those who feel overwhelmed and on edge," says Aviva Romm, MD.

If it's stress that's keeping you awake, reishi can help—it's an "adaptogen," after all, meaning it helps your body to better adapt to the level of stress you're experiencing. Reishi can help you feel calmer, more peaceful, and more grounded and balanced if you're feeling wired or kept awake.

Best Methods of Delivery for Reishi and Sleep:

- Tea, 1 hour before bed, to alleviate stress. You can make tea easily by dissolving reishi powdered extract into hot water.

- Tincture, 30 minutes before bed, taken under the tongue or diluted in a glass of water

- Capsules, taken in the recommended dose on the bottle, 30 minutes before bed

STARLIGHT TONIC

This is a beverage I frequently make as my wind-down drink. Mint tea is calming in the evenings, as it contains no caffeine. All you have to do is add 1 tsp. of your favorite reishi powder and a dropperful of CBD oil at your preferred dosage into your tea (you can use any herbal tea if you don't prefer mint). Try chamomile or lemon balm tea for extra relaxation.

Makes 1 serving

1 tsp. reishi extract powder

1 dropperful of CBD oil (your preferred dosage)

8 oz. mint tea (or other herbal tea of choice)

1 tsp. honey (optional)

Stir reishi and CBD into your mug of hot tea, and sip while winding down in the evening. If you prefer a little bit of sweetness, add honey.

Other Rebel sleep tips:

- Don't drink your tea too close to bedtime (or drink a more concentrated tea with less water, so you aren't waking up to go to the bathroom during the night).

- Get a comfortable sleep mask to block out any light in the room you're sleeping in. I've been using a sleep mask every night for years, and it makes a huge difference.

- Magnesium can be extremely relaxing, and many of us are deficient in it. Take an Epsom salt bath (which is full of magnesium!), make a magnesium tea with powdered magnesium, or take a magnesium capsule. For extra-credit points, find a float tank (sensory-deprivation tank) near you—you'll be floating in magnesium! Book a float in the evening before you head back home to sleep on a day when you're feeling particularly sleep deprived—this is especially helpful for jet lag. Your body will thank you, many times over.

- Use a sound machine—white noise can make a big difference for a sleep-promoting environment, whether the room you're sleeping in is too noisy or too quiet. I have one on the floor next to my bed.

- Watch your intake of alcohol, sugar, and caffeine, especially in the late afternoon and evening. If you're a coffee drinker, consider swapping your afternoon cup for a green tea (green tea naturally contains a calming amino acid called L-theanine, which balances out the caffeine).

- Sleep in a cool room. Studies have shown that between 60 and 67°F is the optimal temperature for sleeping.

- Sleep under a weighted blanket. My sister has a weighted blanket (often referred to as an "anxiety blanket") and every time I visit her I'm amazed at how calming it feels to sleep under it. She recently gifted me one—it relaxes my nervous system and calms me into a deeper sleep.

- Skullcap and passionflower are two herbs known to help with sleep—they can help quiet the mind and stop racing thoughts. You can find these as tinctures or teas. If I wake up in the middle of the night with racing thoughts, taking a tincture of one of these herbs (or another dropperful of CBD oil) can really help coax me back to sleep. Try one at a time to see which one works best for you. A typical dose for an herbal tincture is about 25 drops.

- Try a guided sleep meditation—recently I've gotten into the habit of listening to a guided sleep meditation before I fall asleep, which can help to even further relax the mind. An app called Insight Timer has some great choices.

Anything you can do to lower your overall level of stress and free up some of your energy and mind space during the day (whether it's saying "no" to an event or finding ten or twenty minutes to meditate) can be a huge help when it comes to winding down at night. When you make sleep a priority, other problems may start to melt away. I hope some of these sleep tips will help you find calmness and peace tonight. Sweet dreams!

Rebel Ritual: Swap your nightly glass of wine for reishi tea or a calming herbal tea. If you need something sweet, add a touch of honey.

Terpene Tip: Cannabis varieties high in myrcene (often labeled as "indica" strains) can be extra effective for sleep. If you can find a combination of both myrcene and linalool (the calming terpene in lavender), even better.

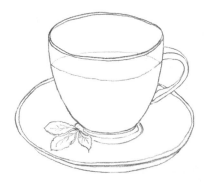

EASE YOUR PAIN

've been a monthly ibuprofen popper since I was twelve years old, when I first started getting menstrual cramps. Whenever I'm at home visiting my parents during the most painful part of my moon cycle, I find myself sneaking into my dad's office in the middle of the night (why do cramps always seem to interrupt us in the middle of the night?) to open his desk drawer and reach into the extra-large Advil bottle he's kept in there *forever*.

Until recently, when the bottle was suddenly gone. This was confusing, as I'd been reaching for that Advil bottle from the exact same drawer for most of my life.

"Dad, what happened to your bottle of Advil?" I asked, after being awake for most of the night in pain with my heating pad. "I couldn't find it last night."

He paused, contemplating. "You know what, Jen? I don't take Advil anymore."

"What?"

"I didn't even realize I stopped taking it. I just don't have any pain anymore."

CANNABIS AND PAIN

Once my dad started on daily CBD oil capsules, his joint pain and arthritis pain vanished. He had no need for over-the-counter pain medicine anymore, which he had taken almost every day for years. We already believed in the benefits of CBD, but it was awesome to witness such a clear before-and-after moment—my dad is now able to walk up and down the stairs with no pain, which was not the case before the CBD (plus, he completely forgot to replenish his lifelong bottle of ibuprofen).

Shortly after this realization, my trusted friend Nicole Jardim, a women's health coach and author of *Fix Your Period,* gave me something to try for my cramps—a CBD/THC vaginal suppository from a company called Foria. I was a little wary, because my cramps were a force to be reckoned with. If something were to actually alleviate the pain, it would be a miracle. Well, as it turns out, miracles tend to happen when cannabis is involved. After inserting the suppository and lying down on the couch to wait, my cramps (which had almost hit their peak pain level of excruciation) started to dissipate. After five minutes, they were substantially less, and after fifteen, they were completely gone. I couldn't believe it. As I started to leave my apartment to head out into New York City (something I'd never normally be doing on the first day of my period), I texted Nicole.

"This thing is incredible. Cramps completely gone in minutes. No joke."

I've been using the suppositories ever since. I had experienced my own before-and-after pain moment with cannabis, just like my dad. Today, neither of us takes ibuprofen (as long as I have cannabis or CBD capsules, topicals, or suppositories on hand). It's pretty wild to say that.

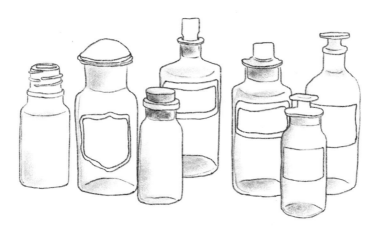

According to a 2018 study, many people taking ibuprofen or other nonsteroidal anti-inflammatory drugs (NSAIDs)—think Advil, Motrin, Aleve, aspirin—are taking more than the recommended dose. These seemingly "safe" over-the-counter drugs make it easy to ignore the label and choose your own dose based on your pain level. Taking NSAIDs has been shown, however, to cause internal bleeding, gastro-intestinal issues, heart attacks, and strokes—and the FDA reports that the risks increase with the dose.

Cannabis has none of these side effects, and as we now know (after becoming experts on the endocannabinoid system), it can actually help to restore our bodies to homeostasis—reducing inflammation and pain.

THE PUBLIC WEIGHS IN ON CANNABIS, OPIOIDS, AND PAIN

In May 2019, the FDA sent out a request for public comments about experiences with CBD. Thousands of people from all over the United States submitted comments, and I read through most of them. The number one thing people mentioned in these comments was pain, with many people reporting that CBD helped them to reduce or eliminate their need for opioids and other pain medications.

"CBD oil allowed my wife to quit opioids and still control her chronic back pain."

"I use CBD daily and it helps decrease my back, neck and hip pain. It also helps to decrease the severity of my daily headaches. I have been able to go from using ten prescription drugs daily to only three."

"I am a disabled veteran and I live in pain every day. Now that I have discovered CBD oil, I've experienced life-changing results and a newfound zest for life. My pain is much more bearable."

"After years of using opiates, I've nearly eliminated them for treating my chronic pain . . . I'm able to add a dose of cannabis in a variety of consumption methods to eliminate pain, or allow me to sleep."

Because we have cannabinoid receptors throughout our bodies, cannabis can help ease many different kinds of pain—including neuropathic pain, headaches, arthritis, fibromyalgia, and inflammatory pain. If you're experiencing pain, here are a few ways cannabis might help:

CANNABIS FOR PAIN RELIEF

- **Quick pain relief.** Inhalation can provide fast relief from pain, and can be combined with a topical, tincture, capsule, or edible to provide long-lasting benefits in addition to the fast-acting relief.

- **Localized pain, headaches, or muscle soreness.** Start with a topical (such as a cream, lotion, salve, or body oil) and massage it into the painful area. For a headache, it can be very soothing to massage a 1:1 CBD-to-THC oil into your temples or the muscles of your neck, depending on where your headache pain originates.

- **Chronic pain, joint pain, arthritis, neuropathic pain, or other pain that is constant.** Try a combination of a topical or transdermal product, and a daily routine of taking a tincture, capsule, or edible, to manage the pain with consistent dosing of cannabinoids.

- **Longer-lasting pain relief.** Capsules and edibles often have better results than tinctures for lasting pain relief, since the effects of using cannabis products orally tend to last longer than using them sublingually. If you have pain throughout the night, try a capsule or edible before bed.

To find your proper dosage for pain with a topical, apply the topical to the painful area, wait fifteen minutes, and see how you feel. If you don't feel any relief, you may need a stronger product or to add more. If you do feel some relief, relax and reapply as needed—the benefits typically last for a few hours.

With tinctures, capsules, or edibles, start with a small dose and work your way up until you find the therapeutic window that provides you with relief. If it's a CBD-only product, you may need to take a higher dose than you would if both CBD and THC are present (as CBD can be more effective in combination with THC).

Many people report greater pain relief from cannabis products that include THC. If you're open to experimenting with higher levels of THC, such as a 1:1 ratio, capsules or edibles can be very effective for pain. Head back to the dosing section on page 69 to learn about experimenting with CBD-to-THC ratios.

CANNABIS FOR MENSTRUAL PAIN

Cannabis has been used for menstrual pain for centuries—it's widely reported that Queen Victoria used a cannabis tincture for her monthly period pain in the 1800s in England—but it's only with the recent discovery of the endocannabinoid system that we are truly beginning to understand how cannabis works to soothe pain. According to Dr. Charles Pollack, the former director of Thomas Jefferson University's Lambert Center for the Study of Medicinal Cannabis and Hemp, the female reproductive tract (in particular, the uterus and lining of the uterus) has an abundance of endocannabinoid receptors, which is why CBD and THC suppositories can provide pain-relieving effects. These suppositories can help with sleep especially during the nights you'd normally wake up with painful cramps.

High-THC products have been found to work extremely well for menstrual pain, but CBD-only products can be highly effective, too. If you use a THC-rich suppository, the THC is being absorbed into the bloodstream, so there's a chance you may feel some psychoactive effects, but most people say they experience deep relaxation, rather than a high. I recommend using the suppositories at night (or during a time when you can relax or take a nap). The effects typically last for a few hours.

If you're feeling experimental, you can make your own CBD or CBD/THC suppositories at home—with only a few ingredients. These suppositories allow you to use higher doses of therapeutic cannabinoids for pain relief without feeling high. For these suppositories, we're using tinctures of CBD oil or a combination of CBD and THC oil. You can play with the dosages based on what's right for you, but I've experienced incredible menstrual pain relief with a 1:1 ratio of CBD to THC. Because we're inserting these suppositories into our bodies, make sure you wash your hands well, use only the highest-quality ingredients, and keep the products clean throughout the process.

QUEEN'S RELIEF SUPPOSITORIES (FOR MENSTRUAL PAIN)

Makes about 10 suppositories, depending on size

½ cup organic cocoa butter

For CBD-only suppositories: 100 mg full-spectrum CBD oil per suppository (divide this by how many suppositories you're making—i.e., 1000 mg total CBD for 10 suppositories)

For CBD/THC combo suppositories: 50 mg THC per suppository, 50 mg CBD per suppository (500 mg THC total for ten suppositories, 500 mg CBD total for ten suppositories)

(These are just general guidelines—you can use whatever amounts you like here, depending on what products you have.)

Suppository molds or tiny silicone ice-cube trays (you can find these online).

Melt the cocoa butter in the top of a double boiler over simmering water on low heat. Stir in the CBD/THC oils until well combined. Be careful not to let the oil or cocoa butter burn.

Pour mixture into suppository molds.

Place in the freezer until solid. Take one out of the freezer whenever that monthly pain starts to creep in! Store in the freezer for up to 6 months.

How to use: Wash your hands, lie down, and insert the suppository into your vagina as you would with a tampon, all the way up to your cervix. Don't worry, it's not freezing, like an ice cube—it's cold, but it will warm up quickly! The cocoa butter will melt once heated by your body, so using these suppositories at bedtime (or when you can lie down for a couple of hours) is suggested.

TOPICALS AND TRANSDERMALS FOR PAIN

For location-specific pain relief (for example, pain from muscle soreness, headaches, or menstrual cramps), a topical cream or lotion can be very soothing. For deeper pain, a transdermal compound or patch penetrates into the tissues and bloodstream, which can provide systematic relief (instead of just local relief). In fact, my tailbone started to hurt while writing this chapter (as I mentioned, I broke my tailbone a few years ago, and writing means sitting for so long!), so I grabbed my 1:1 CBD-to-THC transdermal compound, waited a few minutes, and I couldn't feel the pain anymore.

SOOTHING SALVE

If you're more of a DIY type, here's my favorite at-home recipe for a luxuriously relaxing CBD pain-relief topical salve. In addition to the CBD oil (or THC/CBD oil, if you choose) in this Soothing Salve, I've added lavender and peppermint essential oil for extra pain relief, relaxation, and a cooling effect that works beautifully for pain. As far as dosage goes, you may have to experiment with the dose to see what works for you. Here's a starting point.

Makes 5 ounces

1 oz. shaved beeswax (you can get this online or at a health-food store)

½ cup coconut oil

10 drops lavender essential oil

5 drops peppermint essential oil

100 to 500 mg CBD oil (or a 1:1 CBD-to-THC oil)

Place shaved beeswax in a pan over low heat, pour the oils over top, and melt together.

Once the beeswax and oils have combined, pour the mixture into a jar.

Place your salve in the refrigerator until it solidifies, 10–15 minutes.

Keep at room temperature. If it melts, stir and put in fridge to restore consistency. Rub salve on painful spots on the body as needed.

FREEZER FUDGE "POT BROWNIES"

Okay, we've been talking about edibles for pain, and you're probably wondering when I'm going to get to the real question—when do we get to eat cannabis-infused *chocolate*? Not to worry—I've got you covered.

Combining the magical cannabis plant with mood-boosting, high-quality chocolate may be the best thing you ever did for your pain (especially if it's pain that comes with your monthly cycle!). Here's a delicious way to do it. Let these freezer fudge "pot brownies" ease your pain any time of the month.

These are no-bake "freezer fudge" brownies, which means you can keep them in the freezer and grab one anytime you're in need of a chocolate fix. Feel free to use a higher THC formula here, if you're comfortable with that, for additional pain-relieving effects.

Makes about 10 pieces of fudge, depending on size

1 cup tahini, almond butter, peanut butter, or cashew butter—pick your favorite!

¼ cup coconut oil

¼ cup raw cacao powder

Your desired dosage of full-spectrum CBD oil or CBD/THC oil (if you use 100 mg, each brownie will contain about 10 mg if you have 10 brownies); adjust dosing based on your preference. For flavor, I like to use a mint chocolate CBD oil (from Lazarus Naturals) in this recipe.

¼ cup pure maple syrup

½ tsp. sea salt

1 tsp. vanilla extract

In a medium bowl, whisk together the tahini or nut butter and coconut oil until smooth. If your coconut oil is solid, you may need to heat it slightly in order to whisk it with the nut butter.

Add in the cacao powder, CBD oil, maple syrup, sea salt, and vanilla and stir until smooth and well-combined.

Transfer the mixture to a square or rectangular dish, lined with parchment paper for easy removal.

Place the dish in the freezer and allow it to set for an hour before slicing it up and serving. It will melt if you leave it out too long, so for best results, slice it and then keep it in the freezer, and take out a piece whenever you're ready for a pain-relieving chocolate fix.

MUSHROOMS AND PAIN

While cannabis can provide immediate pain relief, mushrooms often work more behind the scenes to relieve you of pain and inflammation on a more subtle, ongoing basis. All of the medicinal mushrooms in this book have anti-inflammatory properties, which can reduce certain types of pain—but the soothing properties of reishi and the nerve-supporting properties of lion's mane make these two the stars for pain relief.

Anti-Inflammatory Reishi

Reishi mushrooms have powerful anti-inflammatory effects—similar to those of ibuprofen, says Dr. Andrew Weil. Taking reishi daily as a long-term part of your routine can reduce overall inflammation levels in the body. Women who participated in a 2017 study on reishi reported a reduction in fibromyalgia pain after taking 6 g of reishi for 6 weeks. Reishi could be a helpful tool to add to your toolbox, to contribute to lower levels of inflammation in the body and pain reduction. Drink your reishi as a tea, add reishi powder to a smoothie, or take reishi in capsule or tincture form.

Nerve Pain and Lion's Mane

Lion's mane is a worthy addition to your at-home pain regimen if you have any pain related to the nerves. Lion's mane has not only helped my dad manage his chemotherapy-induced neuropathy, but this mushroom can be helpful for people with all varieties of nerve damage or nerve pain, due to the fact that it aids in regenerating the protective myelin sheath around the nerves.

Although lion's mane is a delicious culinary mushroom, if you're taking lion's mane for pain, you will probably want a more concentrated amount of mushroom medicine. A tincture, capsule, or powder extract of lion's mane may be your best bet for nerve pain. Try adding it to your daily regimen for a few weeks and see if your pain lessens.

Other Rebel pain tips:

- **Copaiba.** Many swear by the anti-inflammatory and pain-relieving properties of copaiba essential oil, which contains beta-caryophyllene (the same anti-inflammatory terpene found in some cannabis strains). Mix a few drops into coconut oil and massage into the skin.

- **Turmeric.** Turmeric root is known as one of the most anti-inflammatory foods in the world. The active compound in turmeric—curcumin—can be taken as a supplement, or turmeric can be added as an everyday spice to your meals. It's said that the absorption and effectiveness of turmeric increases by more than 2000 percent when combined with black pepper.

- **Magnesium.** Magnesium is known for decreasing muscle pain and soreness, and many athletes take an Epsom salt bath to soothe sore muscles (Epsom salts are high in magnesium). You can take magnesium as a supplement or apply a magnesium topical product onto sore muscles.

- **Cayenne.** The compound capsaicin in cayenne peppers has anti-inflammatory, detoxifying, and analgesic (pain-relieving) effects and can be added to any food or beverage—as long as you don't mind a little spice.

- **White willow bark.** This is often called "the original aspirin," because it contains a compound called salicin, which has pain-relieving and anti-inflammatory effects. You can find white willow bark in tincture or capsule form.

Rebel Ritual: Next time you find yourself reaching for an ibuprofen or aspirin for joint pain, menstrual pain, a headache, or any other type of everyday pain, try swapping it for a cannabis topical, in combination with a CBD-rich capsule or edible for long-lasting effects. Remember, it may take up to 2 hours for the effects of orally ingested cannabis to kick in.

Terpene Tip: Beta-caryophyllene, also found in black pepper, has been shown to be highly anti-inflammatory. Cannabis strains high in caryophyllene may be extra pain relieving.

Pain is a personal experience that shows up differently for everyone. You will likely have to try a few different methods of pain management before finding what works for you, especially if you're in a habit of taking pain medication.

If you're currently on opioids for pain, please don't attempt to change your dosage or get off of the drugs without your doctor's supervision. If you're hoping to use cannabis to reduce your need for opioids, start slowly and do so under the guidance of your doctor. Dr. Dustin Sulak has a guide to using cannabis to help reduce your need for opioids on his website, Healer.com, and that guide is a great resource to bring to your doctor so you can get started on a reasonable plan together.

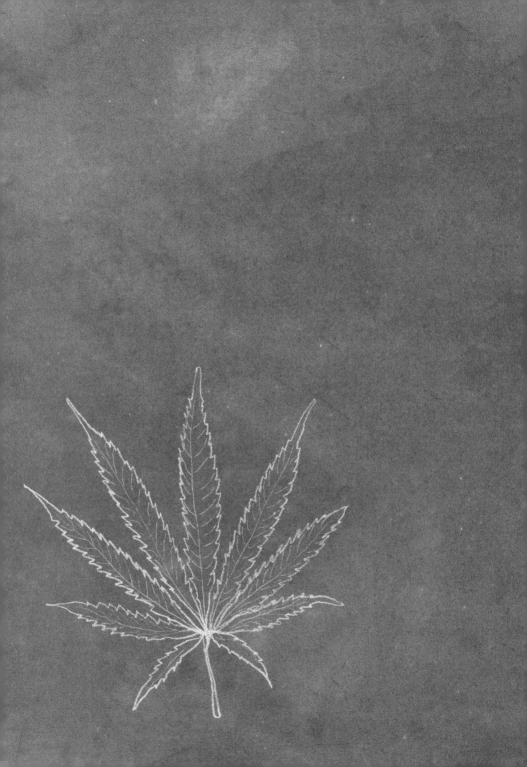

CALM STRESS AND ANXIETY

Stress and anxiety are rampant epidemics these days. We're constantly bombarded with stimulation of all kinds. With technology advancing at such a fast pace, our brains need to work overtime to catch up. We're hooked on social media, glued to artificial light, and under constant pressure to produce, achieve, and succeed. Life feels like it's moving at lightning speed—and we all have way too many tabs open in our brains. I live in New York City (appropriately nicknamed "the city that never sleeps"), so that stress and anxiety are especially obvious here, but of course it's happening everywhere. Our nervous systems are constantly in fight-or-flight mode—making it hard to sleep, relax, breathe, smile, be present, and enjoy life.

The way we're encouraged to handle stress and anxiety isn't helping the issue. Alcohol, sugar, prescription drugs, endless surfing of the Internet—we turn to these things to help take the edge off, which puts us in a constant cycle of self-medicating. This creates even *more* anxiety and stress in our bodies and in our minds.

OUR BODIES ARE PRACTICALLY
BEGGING US TO SLOW DOWN.

We need to be nurtured and nourished, and our nervous systems need to be settled.

The good news is, cannabis and mushrooms can both be used to support the nervous system and to calm anxiety and stress, and if you add the right plants, herbs, and fungi to your apothecary, you'll be on your way to feeling more at ease and able to show up for your life with more presence and joy.

A note on medications: As I mentioned at the beginning of the book, "natural" or "herbal" does not always mean "better." If you need or want to be on medication for anxiety, do what works best for you, take care of your body and mind as well as you can, and work with a therapist to get the support you need. None of these recommendations should be considered alternatives to your doctor-prescribed anxiety medication.

CANNABIS AND ANXIETY

I was surprised when I first tried CBD—I could physically feel it calming my anxiety. For me, anxiety often feels like tightness in my chest and racing thoughts (when I'm trying to fall asleep, of course), and the first time I took CBD oil, I could feel that physical "sharpness" smooth out. I was able to relax into sleep without feeling anxious. It was subtle and extraordinary at the same time.

Anxiety is correlated with low levels of the endocannabinoid anandamide in the brain, and taking CBD increases our natural levels of anandamide. This points us to why CBD may be so effective in reducing anxiety. Anxiety is one of the top things people report feeling relief from when using CBD. I frequently get emails like this one:

> Jenny, CBD has changed my life. It has helped with anxiety
> (this is huge for me!), better sleep, zero sore muscles after
> hard workouts, and better digestion. I use a full-spectrum
> tincture, which I prefer. I take it once per day at bedtime.
> I can't say enough about how surprised and amazed I am—
> it has helped me way more than anti-anxiety meds. I'm not
> against meds, but CBD oil works better for me.

CBD OR THC FOR ANXIETY?

High-CBD products are often preferred over high-THC products for easing anxiety, as THC can be anxiety-promoting for some. If you struggle with anxiety, you will likely want to try a product with a higher ratio of CBD to THC (18:1 or higher could be a good place to start), although self-experimentation is key. I get a lot of relief from anxiety with high-CBD products (the "hemp-based" CBD oils with .3 percent THC or less) along with CBD-to-THC ratios of 20:1 or 30:1. If you do decide to experiment with a higher-THC product, remember to start very low and use just enough to find relief from your anxiety without feeling uncomfortable. As far as dosing goes, you may find you need less CBD during the day to calm your anxiety in order to stay focused and alert—and more CBD at night when it's time to wind down.

Best Methods of Delivery for Stress and Anxiety

- **Immediate relief: inhalation.** Inhalation has the quickest onset time of all delivery methods, which means the antianxiety effects are fast acting. Of course, smoking and vaporizing both come with drawbacks (including the chemicals in the smoke, respiratory irritation, and the potentially harmful chemicals found in some vape cartridges), so if you choose to go the inhalation route, try an herbal vaporizer (which heats the compounds in the cannabis to the point where you can benefit from the cannabinoids and terpenes, but doesn't combust or burn the plant material, or create smoke).

- **Quick relief of anxiety and stress: tincture.** Instead of immediate effects, an oil tincture under the tongue will kick in after about 15 minutes and last a bit longer than the effects of inhalation. Try a few drops of CBD oil under the tongue, then wait 15 minutes to see how you feel before taking more. You may be surprised to feel your anxiety calming down quickly.

- **Long-lasting relief: capsule or edible.** These methods of consuming CBD that go through your digestive system can be helpful if you want something long-lasting, but keep in mind that the onset won't be as quick. If you're dealing with acute anxiety and want to feel calmed right away, taking a tincture or inhalation in addition to a capsule or edible might be the best bet—as a capsule or edible could take up to 2 hours to have an effect.

- **General stress relief: topical.** While body oil isn't typically the quickest method of delivery for calming anxiety, your skin is covered with cannabinoid receptors—so lathering on a CBD-rich (or THC-rich) body oil, especially right after a hot shower, can be extremely calming and stress reducing. Try it at night to calm anxiety before sleep. I love the Apothecanna brand for cannabis body oils.

MUSHROOMS AND ANXIETY

One of the greatest known medicinal mushrooms for stress and anxiety is reishi. Reishi acts as an adaptogen, helping your body to better "adapt" to the stressors in your life. Not only that, but taking reishi can support your adrenals, which can have a calming effect and help lower your stress. A 2011 study with breast cancer patients showed that participants reported lowered anxiety and depression and a better overall sense of well-being after using reishi for four weeks.

"It is little surprise that reishi is so effective as a calmative, helping alleviate anxiety, insomnia, and nervousness associated with adrenal deficit conditions," says Robert Rogers in *The Fungal Pharmacy*. "It helps relax muscles and reduces the effect of caffeine on the body."

It's said that the Shaolin monks have used reishi for centuries, to help them achieve deeper meditations—reishi tea and meditation could be a wonderfully calming ritual to add to your evening routine.

Lion's mane has also been shown to help with anxiety and depression, as it supports brain health. A 2018 study in mice showed that an extract of lion's mane reduced anxiety by promoting neurogenesis (the formation of new neurons) in the brain.

Chaga can also help regulate the body's response to stress, and it can have a grounding effect when you're feeling anxious.

A combination of lion's mane, chaga, and reishi mushrooms could be a great daily tonic for your nerves. I have tinctures of all three in my kitchen, along with powder extracts to mix into hot water for teas. I take a tincture or drink a cup of powdered extract in hot water whenever I need to ease my nerves.

Methods of Delivery for Stress and Anxiety

- **Calm your nerves: tea.** Try swapping out your coffee (the caffeine could be adding to your anxiety) for a mug of hot mushroom tea. You can steep dried reishi slices or chunks of chaga in hot water, or keep it simple with a reishi, chaga, or lion's mane extract powder that you can dissolve into hot water. The ritual of making and drinking the tea will help soothe your nerves, and it's also a nice swap if you usually drink a glass of wine to relax. It may take some getting used to if you're a regular alcohol drinker, to start drinking a calming tea instead, but try it a few times—you may just fall in love with the feeling!

- **Feel relaxed and grounded: tincture or capsule.** Add a tincture or capsule of reishi, chaga, and lion's mane into your routine. Take 1–2 dropperfuls of a tincture per day in water, tea, or straight into your mouth. Do this daily, and you will feel your stress and anxiety lift as you feel more grounded and your nervous system begins to relax. Because these mushrooms work subtly, it may take you a week or two to really notice that you're feeling more relaxed and grounded as you go about your day-to-day life.

Other Rebel stress and anxiety tips:

- **Oat straw.** Oat straw is known by herbalists as a daily tonic for the nervous system. You can drink oat straw tea at any time of day (it's neither stimulating or sedating) or make an oat straw infusion, which is similar to tea except you let it steep overnight, creating a stronger and more nutritionally potent brew.

- **Lemon balm.** Lemon balm is another wonderful calming herb that's soothing to drink as a tea during the day or at night. I find lemon balm tea to be particularly nourishing in the early evening as I'm transitioning from the activity of the day into the calmness of night.

- **Tulsi (holy basil).** Tulsi is a prominent herb in Ayurvedic medicine and has been used for thousands of years as an antidote to stress. You can find tulsi in tea or take it in capsules or tinctures.

- **Ashwagandha.** Ashwagandha is a medicinal herb that is widely known for stress reduction and nervous system support. Studies have shown that taking 500–600 mg of ashwagandha per day can lower anxiety levels. You can add ashwagandha powder to smoothies, drink it as a tea, or take capsules or tinctures.

- **Breathwork.** Learning to calm anxiety with breathwork may be one of the most powerful tools we have in our toolbelt (plus, breathing is free!). Dr. Andrew Weil's 4-7-8 Breath is one of the easiest and most effective. You breathe in through your nose for a count of 4, hold your breath for a count of 7, and breathe out through your nose for a count of 8. Do this four times, and then continue as many times as you need to until you feel calm.

- **Restorative yoga.** Restorative yoga poses can be incredibly calming to the nervous system. One of the easiest and most calming restorative poses is "legs up the wall." It's exactly what it sounds like—lie down with your back on the floor or bed and put your legs up the wall. Stay this way for 25 breaths. This is a good practice if you find yourself too wound up to relax.

- **Meditation.** Any kind of meditation practice can help tremendously with lowering anxiety levels. If you're new to meditation, try listening to a guided meditation through an app

(Headspace and Insight Timer are both wonderful), or simply sit for 10 minutes and focus on your inhale and your exhale.

- **Float tanks.** Sensory-deprivation tanks are one of my personal favorite ways to treat myself to the ultimate hour of stress relief. In a float tank, you can quickly be taken into a state of deep relaxation and meditation, while soaking in 800 pounds of Epsom salt (which is high in calming magnesium). If you've never tried a float tank, do a search to see if there's one near you, and experience the ultimate feeling of quietude.

Rebel Ritual: Purposefully take some time to incorporate stress-reducing practices into your everyday life, particularly if you're always on the go. Take a few moments after your shower to intentionally massage a soothing cannabis body oil into your skin, sip on reishi tea in the afternoon or evening, pause throughout your day to take a few deep breaths, or go for a walk in nature.

Terpene Tip: Cannabis varieties high in the terpene linalool (found in lavender) tend to be especially soothing for anxiety. If you want some extra linalool in your life, get some lavender essential oil and use it in a diffuser in your home or office for a dose of calm.

STRESS-MELTING BODY OIL

¼ cup carrier oil—(I like almond oil, jojoba oil, or fractionated coconut oil which is liquid rather than solid)

1 dropperful of a CBD or CBD/THC tincture

A few drops of a calming essential oil, such as lavender or rose

In a bowl, add desired amount of unflavored CBD/THC tincture to the carrier oil (alternatively, you can use your infused coconut oil that you made with the cannabis flower).

Add a few drops of your favorite essential oil—such as lavender or rose.

Whisk all oils together well and put mixture into a glass bottle with a pump.

Use on your body as a massage oil, whenever you're in need of stress relief.

HEALTHY CBD GUMMIES

CONTRIBUTED BY ROBYN YOUKILIS

One of the top reasons people are reaching for CBD gummies is relaxation and taming anxiety, but most CBD gummies on the market today contain sugar, corn syrup, artificial colors, and artificial flavors. My friend Robyn Youkilis has an amazing healthy gummy recipe in her book *Go With Your Gut* (it's called "Good Gut Gummies" because of the gut-friendly gelatin). Here, we've joined forces to create healthier CBD gummies, sweetened with honey and made with real fruit. The main recipe uses blueberries, but Robyn offers yummy alternatives like strawberry, raspberry, and peach. True to form, I've added my own energy-boosting flavor ideas—coffee gummies and matcha gummies. The possibilities are endless!

Servings depend on size and cut

1 cup frozen blueberries or raspberries
(or a mix of the two)

¾ cup fresh lemon or lime juice
(or a mix of the two)

1 Tbsp. honey

¼ cup unflavored Great Lakes
Gelatin

2–3 dropperfuls of full-spectrum CBD oil, depending on your
desired dose—I make mine with 10–20mg of CBD per gummy. Take
note of total amount of milligrams you add, so you can measure
individual serving sizes.

Add the berries to a small saucepan over medium heat.

Stir the berries and allow them to cook until their released liquid
is steaming and the berries are plump, 6–10 minutes.

Place the lemon juice, honey, and berries into a high-speed
blender or food processor and blend until smooth. Remove the
lid and allow the mixture to cool slightly.

Add the gelatin and CBD oil to the blender and blend again until
smooth.

Pour the mixture into candy molds, or a 9x9-inch baking dish,
and refrigerate for 30 minutes to 1 hour.

Once the gummies have set, remove them from the molds or
slice them into desired shapes and store in the refrigerator.

Cut into small pieces depending on your desired dose (if you
want each gummy to have 10 mg of CBD and you started with
100 mg, you will cut 10 squares, for example).

If you want a no-sugar version, you can try sweetening with monk fruit sweetener or stevia, if you like the taste.

OTHER FLAVORS TO TRY:

Peach (add peaches instead of blueberries)

Strawberry (add strawberries instead of blueberries)

Matcha: warm 1 cup coconut milk with 2 tsp. matcha, add to blender with gelatin, 2 Tbsp. honey, and CBD—no lemon juice

Coffee: warm ½ cup coffee and ½ cup coconut milk, add to blender with gelatin, 2 Tbsp. honey, and CBD—no lemon juice

EVENING ADAPTOGENIC ELIXIR

CONTRIBUTED BY JAMIE GRABER

My friend Jamie Graber—of Organically, Jamie—once owned a juice shop in the West Village of NYC, where she made all kinds of wonderful juices, smoothies, coffee drinks, and elixirs. She's a master at beverage-making, especially using health-supportive adaptogens. She's contributed both a morning and evening elixir to *The Rebel's Apothecary*. This is the evening elixir, which includes both CBD and soothing reishi and is perfect for calming stress and anxiety. (You can find Jamie's energizing morning elixir on page 217!)

10–12 oz. warm water

¼–½ tsp. reishi extract powder

¼–½ tsp. ashwagandha powder

¼—½ tsp. cinnamon

1 dropperful of CBD oil (your preferred evening dose)

½—1 tsp. ghee or coconut oil

Put the warm liquid into a blender, and then add the rest of the ingredients. It should be tea temperature—warm to the touch, not scalding. Blend, pour into a mug, and sip.

Jamie and I both prefer our elixirs to taste earthy and medicinal—but if you want some added sweetness, add a touch of honey, stevia, or your sweetener of choice.

INCREASE YOUR ENERGY, ENHANCE YOUR FOCUS, UPLIFT YOUR MOOD

ENERGY

Thas a time in my life when my preferred methods for boosting my energy throughout the day were Adderall, cocaine, and multiple extra-large iced coffees with three packets of artificial sweetener in each one. Those were not my proudest days, and they came with major downfalls—one being severe energy crashes. One thing that was glaringly obvious about my stimulant habit: I was always looking for quick energy. I was depleted, exhausted, constantly self-medicating, and dipping well below the reserves of my energy in order to make it through the day. I felt like a slave to those stimulants, because if I didn't take them, I couldn't keep my eyes open at work.

While I still love my espresso, and I'll likely always be drawn to energy boosters, I reach for healthier alternatives now. Instead of reaching for artificial sources of energy all day long, I'm much more mindful about how the foods I eat, the beverages I drink, and my overall life-style affect my energy.

So many of us struggle with energy on a day-to-day basis, and it can feel like a never-ending spiral of peaks and crashes. While cannabis and mushrooms can be nourishing and supportive, it's important that your diet and lifestyle are supporting you, too. Taking care of your body and mind requires a holistic approach, and if you struggle with low energy, it's likely going to require some lifestyle shifts. The great thing about cannabis and mushrooms is that when they're used mindfully and in the right ways, in tandem with a healthy lifestyle, they can support and nourish your body and mind to help you enhance and sustain your natural energy.

FOCUS

In this world of overstimulation, being able to focus and be present with our work and our creative projects has become increasingly difficult. People today report having less ability to concentrate than ever before, as our attention is constantly being pulled in a million different directions. Social media doesn't help—the endless notifications, scrolling through thousands of photos and updates about other people's lives, and the pressure to constantly share deflects our focus from the projects we really want to (and need to) be working on. Imagine what we could accomplish if we were truly able to focus our attention and brainpower on the creative projects we're most passionate about. The world doesn't make it easy. In fact, in order to write this book, I had to get off of social media completely. As I began writing, I could sense that social media was pulling my attention in ways that were distracting me from the hours of dedicated focus that writing a book truly requires.

Setting boundaries with distractions such as social media, the Internet, mindless entertainment, and even people can be an important place to start when it comes to increasing your focus. Getting clear about your priorities and values and what you really want to focus on is the first step. Once you're clear on your priorities, you can call in your plant and fungi friends to give you a little brain boost to enhance your creative productivity.

When it comes to the brain, both cannabis and medicinal mushrooms have been shown to promote neurogenesis—the process by which new neurons are formed in the brain—and to have neuroprotective effects. Research has widely shown that the formation of new neurons (particularly in the brain's hippocampus) 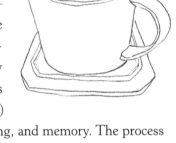 contributes to cognitive function, learning, and memory. The process of neurogenesis becomes increasingly important as we age, to keep us sharp and focused. As it turns out, both cannabis and mushrooms can play a key role in keeping our brainpower in tip-top shape.

MOOD

"Mood" can be a general term that describes feelings of ease, joy, or wellness—but it can also refer to more serious issues of depression or other mental health struggles. There's a wide range of variations when it comes to the word "mood," but in this section we're covering how cannabis and mushrooms can support gentle mood elevation. If you struggle with severe depression or any other mental health issue, diet and lifestyle changes can be hugely beneficial to your overall well-being, but please work with your doctor or psychiatrist to come up with a treatment plan.

Speaking of depression, later in this book we'll cover some of the current research on psilocybin mushrooms (the psychedelic ones) and treatment-resistant depression. While this research is still emerging, the results have been really exciting so far and psilocybin mushrooms could truly become a game-changer for people suffering with depression.

That being said, cannabis and some of the non-psychedelic medicinal mushrooms can be very supportive for enhancing mood. The endocannabinoid system (which cannabis interacts with) is highly tied in with mood—as you know, anandamide, one of our endogenous (inner) cannabinoids, is associated with the euphoria of a runner's high. Depression has also been linked to low levels of the endocannabinoid 2-AG. Our CB1 receptors play a huge role in mood regulation, and it's been shown that blocking the CB1 receptors can cause major depressive episodes. More research needs to be done here, but many people report improved mood through the use of cannabis.

CANNABIS FOR ENERGY, FOCUS, AND MOOD

When I first met Greg Prasker, one of the founders of SupHERBals CBD oil (the first CBD oil I tried, and one that I still use to this day), I had been taking CBD for anxiety and sleep for a few months. When I asked him what he used CBD for most often, he said, "I take it in the morning and it really helps me with focus." I was surprised to hear that, given that I had been using it only in the evenings, to help me chill out. "Taking it in smaller amounts during the day really helps me concentrate on work," he explained. He's not the only one—I've heard many reports from people that taking small amounts of CBD throughout the day can be stimulating and wake-promoting, rather than sedating, and can provide a welcome boost to focus, energy, and mood.

Methods of Delivery for Energy, Focus, and Mood:

- **Smaller doses of CBD** are often reported to work best for focus, concentration, mood, energy, and general daytime use, as higher doses can make some people feel sleepy. Just a few drops—5 mg may be a good place to start, but you may need a little less or a little more. Start low and see how you feel after 15 minutes. Don't take too much at once if you're about to sit down for a full day of meetings on a busy workday. Experiment with your dosing on a lower-stakes day.

- **Inhalation**—While tinctures can provide more accurate dosing, inhalation can provide a quick boost of focus, creativity, and mood enhancement. Researchers from Washington State University found that adults reported a reduction in depressive symptoms with just one puff of high-CBD, low-THC medical cannabis.

- **Microdoses of THC** (1–2 mg, or even less) are sometimes used for focus, mood, and concentration, but tread wisely, as taking just a *little* bit too much THC can impair focus and cause anxiety in some. If you want to experiment with microdosing THC for focus and mood, I *definitely* recommend trying it on a low-stakes day—not a day where you have to give a presentation or have a big meeting or deadline. Taking microdoses of THC can be easily measured with a tincture—try one drop (one drop only!) under your tongue and wait 15 minutes. Remember, THC is more potent than CBD and it's much easier to take more later if you need to, rather than backtrack if you've taken too much.

MUSHROOMS FOR ENERGY, FOCUS, AND MOOD

Mushrooms are superstars for brain power—particularly lion's mane. Studies on lion's mane and the active compounds within it (called hericenones and erinacines) show that it can induce NGF, or nerve growth factor synthesis in nerve cells. This is one of the reasons lion's mane has been known to help with neuropathy, by regenerating the myelin sheath (or protective coating) around damaged nerves. As lion's mane has been shown in studies to support and improve cognitive function, people are using it to get through a focused workday with great results. I've stayed up writing on many late nights with a warm mug of lion's mane tea. Lion's mane has also been shown to reduce anxiety and depression, so it could give you a mood boost, too!

Cordyceps is widely acclaimed as the "energy mushroom," as it increases blood flow and oxygen circulation in the body, and has been shown to increase ATP, which can enhance energy and reduce fatigue. Studies in animal models have also shown that the cordyceps mushroom can improve learning and memory and have neuroprotective effects, so it can't hurt to add it to the focus and brain power arsenal, too. Lion's mane and cordyceps together may just be the perfect combination for boosting mood, energy, and brainpower.

Methods of Delivery for Energy, Focus, and Mood:

- **Lion's mane.** Add lion's mane powder to your daily coffee, tea, or smoothie. You can also take lion's mane as a tincture or capsule to help you with focusing and mood enhancement.

- **Cordyceps.** Athletes commonly take cordyceps for energy and stamina before a workout. Mix cordyceps powder into your morning beverage, or combine cordyceps with lion's mane in a smoothie to get an extra boost of energy and brain power. As with lion's mane, you can also take cordyceps in tincture or capsule form.

- **Microdoses of psilocybin.** Psilocybin (the psychedelic compound in magic mushrooms) is currently illegal, so this is for informational purposes only, but there's a reason "microdosing"—taking tiny, sub-perceptual amounts—of magic mushrooms has become so popular. One of the most frequently touted benefits of microdosing with psilocybin is that it can lift depression, sharpen focus, and enhance creativity. More studies are being conducted as we speak, and as legality shifts and psilocybin becomes legal for use therapeutically, you can expect more doctors to become versed in the benefits. Head to RebelsApothecary.com/Resources for the latest updates on psilocybin research. Find more on psilocybin microdosing on page 312.

Other Rebel tips for energy, focus, and mood

- **Matcha tea.** The health benefits of matcha (powdered green tea) have been known for thousands of years. Matcha can help to promote mental clarity, elevation in mood, and enhanced energy, making it the perfect alternative to coffee. Matcha contains L-theanine, which is relaxing, along with caffeine, which contributes to a well-rounded and calming energy. A recipe for preparing the perfect bowl of matcha and an adaptogenic matcha cold brew are coming up next in this section, from Dr. Andrew Weil and Matcha Kari.

- **Yerba mate tea.** The first time I tried a hot mug of yerba mate tea (from the yerba mate tree, native to South America), I knew I had found my favorite way to consume caffeine. The energy-boosting, mood-lifting, and focus-enhancing properties of yerba mate tea are well documented, and it's been shown to support a healthy metabolism.

- **Fermented foods.** They say our gut is our "second brain" and that nourishing the balance of our gut flora can be crucial for mood and brain power. Fermented foods such as sauerkraut and kombucha or taking a probiotics supplement can be supportive to the gut and, therefore, the brain.

- **Healthy fats.** Some of these include coconut oil, MCT oil, and omega-3 fish oils, which can help to nourish your brain and keep you feeling energized and sharp.

- **L-tyrosine.** This is an amino acid, and I've found it to be an all-star in my life for focus, energy, and mood. I recommend reading *The Mood Cure* by Julia Ross for great information on amino-acid therapy and which amino acids might work for you.

- **Nootropics.** A nootropic is a dietary supplement that can support brain function. One I particularly like is called Alpha Brain from Onnit (it contains both L-tyrosine, which I mentioned above, and L-theanine, found in green tea).

- **Water.** Yes, water! I know this sounds too simple to be true, but dehydration can be a major cause of low energy. Next time your energy dips, try a cold glass of water instead of something caffeinated.

Rebel Ritual: One of the energy, mood, and focus tricks I used while writing this book was to combine lion's mane extract with yerba mate tea. I find it to be mentally stimulating and uplifting in a more sustainable way than coffee. Mixing a teaspoon of lion's mane powder into a hot mug of yerba mate made for many long afternoons of writing and researching. I'll also make this elixir to boost my energy and mood if I'm getting ready to go to a social event (as I don't drink alcohol). Lion's mane plus yerba mate tea can boost energy, mood, and focus all at once.

FOCUS ELIXIR

1 tsp. lion's mane powder per mug of tea

1 pot of hot yerba mate tea (I use loose-leaf yerba mate tea prepared in a French press)

Stir the lion's mane powder into your hot yerba mate for powerful focused energy and an uplifting mood boost.

Terpene Tip for focus: Cannabis varieties high in pinene (also found in pine needles and pine nuts) can help with mental clarity and focus. In fact, because it's alerting and promotes memory retention, pinene can help to reduce the brain fogginess you might experience from taking too much THC. You can also eat pine nuts or inhale the scent of fresh pine (take a walk through a pine-tree forest for the ultimate pinene experience).

Terpene Tip for mood and energy: Cannabis varieties that are high in limonene (found in citrus fruits) are known to produce antidepressant and energy-boosting effects. Inhaling the scent of lemon or orange (either the actual fruit or diffused essential oils) can help to uplift you. For the ultimate daytime cannabis experience, ask your budtender to recommend a CBD-rich variety that has both limonene and pinene present—these terps are often associated with "sativa" strains.

HOW TO BREW THE PERFECT BOWL OF MATCHA

CONTRIBUTED BY DR. ANDREW WEIL AND MATCHA KARI

I've mentioned Dr. Andrew Weil quite a few times in this book, as he's one of the pioneers of holistic and integrative medicine—especially when it comes to medicinal mushrooms! I've followed his work for many years, so when I found out he started his own matcha tea company called Matcha Kari, I ordered some immediately. I'm so thrilled that Dr. Weil and Matcha Kari have contributed these recipes to *The Rebel's Apothecary*—first, instructions for brewing the perfect bowl of matcha, and second, an adaptogenic matcha "cold brew." Enjoy the calm, focused energy!

Makes 1 serving

1 cup hot water

1 tsp. sifted matcha powder

Heat water in a kettle until steam first appears; this will be well below boiling, about 180°F.

Turn off heat.

Pour about ½ cup of hot water into a matcha bowl (a small ceramic bowl) to warm it; discard the water and dry the inside of the bowl.

Place the matcha powder in the warmed bowl.

Add about ¼ cup (2 oz.) of hot water to the matcha in the bowl.

Use a tea whisk to mix the matcha tea into the water. Begin with a slow, back-and-forth stroke, then bring the mixture to a froth with quick strokes.

Sip and enjoy.

ADAPTOGENIC MATCHA COLD BREW

CONTRIBUTED BY DR. ANDREW WEIL AND MATCHA KARI

Typically, Dr. Weil drinks his matcha 100 percent plain, though he's a huge fan of cold-brew style. In this recipe, he offers a few options for adding adaptogens to a cold matcha tea. I love the taste and quality of the matcha from Matcha Kari, available online.

There's a lot to choose from, so it's important to wisely consider taste and *especially* quality when crafting an Adaptogenic Matcha Cold Brew. Importantly, the final appearance should carry a sense of wise choice and the minimal use of adaptogens to accent, not mask the flavor of the matcha—while also getting an extra health boost.

—*Dr. Andrew Weil*

Makes one 12-oz. serving

1–2 tsp. matcha powder

Choose *only* one or two of these time-tested adaptogenic herbs, roots, or mushrooms:

2–3 tsp. fresh juice (or ¼ tsp. powder) from

Ashwagandha

Ginger

Turmeric

Mushroom tincture (or ¼ tsp. powder) from favorites such as:

Reishi

Cordyceps

Maitake

Lion's mane

Add about ¾ cup of ice to a 12-oz. drinking glass; set aside.

With an 8-oz. mixing cup, use a bamboo whisk (alternatively, an electric frother) to mix together 1–2 tsp. matcha with any powders mentioned above, and 6 oz. of room-temperature water.

Once powders are fully dissolved in the water, add any fresh juices or tinctures mentioned above and gently swirl.

Finally, pour over ice in the glass you set aside, and enjoy!

MORNING ADAPTOGENIC ELIXIR

CONTRIBUTED BY JAMIE GRABER
OF ORGANICALLY, JAMIE

You've already seen Jamie's evening elixir (on page 203), and this is her energizing morning version. Making morning coffee drinks with supportive herbal add-ins is one of my favorite self-care rituals. This one combines espresso with our beloved cordyceps, and adds maca—an adaptogenic root known to enhance energy and stamina. As with the evening elixir, you can add a dash of your favorite sweetener if you prefer (although maca provides a slightly subtle sweetness). Talk about a nourishing upgrade to your morning coffee!

Makes 1 serving

2 shots espresso

8 oz. warm water (or 1 cup brewed coffee, in place of espresso and water)

¼–½ tsp. cordyceps powder

1 tsp. maca powder

¼–½ tsp. cinnamon

½–1 tsp. ghee or coconut oil

Put the warm liquid into a blender, and then add the rest of the ingredients. It should be tea temperature—warm to the touch, not scalding.

Blend all ingredients in blender.

If you don't drink coffee, you can sub it out for plain water, matcha, or another tea. You can easily add lion's mane to this recipe too, for even more of an uplifting boost!

REBEL'S GREEN JUICE

This green juice recipe with CBD always gives me an energy and mood boost—I especially love drinking it when I'm inclined to reach for yet another coffee. The juice hydrates and sends nutrition to my cells and always leaves me feeling better than before. I prefer my green juices without fruit, but if you want an extra kick of sweetness, you can add an apple or pear to this recipe.

Makes 1 serving

1 cucumber

2–4 celery stalks

1 lime

1 lemon

1-inch piece of ginger

Small dose of your favorite CBD oil (I use 5-10mg for daytime).

Optional additional herb add-ins: basil, cilantro, or mint to taste

Juice cucumber, celery, lime, lemon, and ginger in a juicer. Add optional ingredients. Add the juice to a blender with CBD oil and blend, or add to a shaker bottle and shake to combine the CBD with the juice. If you don't have a juicer, you can get your favorite green juice from a juice shop, pour it into a shaker bottle, add your favorite CBD oil, and shake.

CORDYCEPS ENERGY BARS

CONTRIBUTED BY OLGA COTTER
OF MUSHROOM MOUNTAIN

When I took a medicinal mushroom seminar with mycologist Tradd Cotter at the Mushroom Mountain research facility in South Carolina, his wife, Olga, made us the most delicious Cordyceps Energy Bars to snack on throughout the day. Packed with cordyceps extract, they are perfect as an energy-boosting snack or breakfast, or to take with you for stamina on a long hike.

Makes about 12 bars

1 cup powdered oats

3 Tbsp. cacao powder

¾ cup crunchy almond butter, cashew butter, or peanut butter (choose your favorite)

2 Tbsps. cordyceps extract powder

½ cup protein powder (I like organic whey, hemp, or pea protein)

1 cup dates or figs, chopped

¼ cup dark chocolate chips

½ cup pure maple syrup

Add all ingredients to a bowl and mix well—or use a food processor to get a smoother consistency. Add mixture to rectangular 8x8-inch baking dish (or similar), and put in fridge for 30 minutes before cutting into bars.

REBEL'S COFFEE

This CBD and mushroom coffee is one of my go-to morning staples. I combine a mushroom blend powder with mint chocolate CBD oil, and add it to my regular morning coffee. Although some question the validity of using CBD and coffee in combination, I love the feeling—using a small dose of CBD takes the edge off of the caffeine, provides a little mood boost, and helps me to focus.

2 shots espresso with 1 cup water (or 1 cup regular coffee)

1 tsp. mushroom blend powder (I love the mushroom blends from Four Sigmatic or SuperFeast)

1 dropperful of mint chocolate CBD oil (I like Lazarus Naturals or Charlotte's Web—choose your daytime dosage—I use 5–10mg)

Your creamer of choice (I like a coconut/almond milk blend, Nutpods brand)

Use a spoon to mix all ingredients in a mug—or blend in a blender to better mix the CBD oil into the liquid.

UPGRADE YOUR IMMUNITY

The human immune system is a complex balancing act. When we have an infection or disease to fight, our immune system "upregulates," or becomes stronger, to fight the infection and bring us back into balance. Too much immune activity, however, can lead to an overactive immune system—which is the case in autoimmune conditions. Cannabis and medicinal mushrooms have both been shown to have immunomodulating effects, meaning they help keep the immune system in balance—stimulating it when there's something to fight (such as cancer) and downregulating it when it's overactive (in the case of autoimmune conditions). Mushrooms, in particular, have immune-supporting properties across the board. Of course, cannabis and mushrooms may not be right for your particular condition—so when dealing with a serious illness or diagnosis, work with your doctor to figure out the right treatment plan for you.

CANNABIS AND THE IMMUNE SYSTEM

Our endocannabinoid system plays a major role in keeping our immune system in balance. We have cannabinoid receptors located throughout the immune system (both CB1 and CB2, with CB2 being more abundant), which help to regulate inflammation (our body's natural response to injury or infection). Our immune system controls everything from fighting off the common cold to warding off serious disease.

According to a 2009 study published in *Pharmacological Research,* our endocannabinoids (anandamide and 2-AG) are potent immunomodulators and play a role in regulating many different kinds of immune cells—including T cells, B cells, lymphocytes, macrophages, and natural killer cells (which are responsible for defending against cancer). Anandamide and 2-AG have both been shown to slow tumor growth and induce apoptosis (or cell death) of cancer cells. This same study suggests that delaying the breakdown of our natural endocannabinoids (which CBD does) could be a novel therapeutic treatment against inflammatory and autoimmune diseases.

Therefore, making sure our endocannabinoid system is properly nourished—by adding in phytocannabinoids from cannabis to support it—can play a key role in keeping our immune system strong, preventing disease, and staying healthy.

How to use cannabis for immune support:

- **Take a full-spectrum CBD-rich tincture.** Because the immune system is such a delicate balance, and research is still being done on the immunomodulating effects of cannabis, it may be helpful to take a full-spectrum CBD oil tincture as a daily tonic for the endocannabinoid system. A daily "tonic" means that something tonifies your system, bringing consistent balance, restoration, and daily support without being overly stimulating or sedating. A full-spectrum product gives you access to a wide range of phytocannabinoids from the cannabis plant, each playing a role in supporting the endocannabinoid system and preventing the breakdown of our natural endocannabinoids. Think of this as a daily multivitamin to help keep you healthy and in harmony. I take a dropperful of a full-spectrum CBD tincture every night before I wind down for bed.

MUSHROOMS AND THE IMMUNE SYSTEM

Helping to regulate the immune system is one of the greatest known superpowers of all medicinal mushrooms. Every medicinal mushroom covered in *The Rebel's Apothecary* has been shown in studies to have potent immunomodulating effects, and mushrooms have been celebrated as immune enhancers throughout all of history.

As we learned in the mushroom section, all medicinal mushrooms contain powerful polysaccharides called beta-glucans, which have been found to help fight inflammation and balance the immune system.

"Beta glucans attach themselves to the receptor sites on the immune cells and activate them, allowing them to recognize cancer cells as 'foreign' and create a higher level of response," says Robert Rogers in *The Fungal Pharmacy*.

It's tough to pick one medicinal mushroom as the most powerful for immunity—they all have tremendous benefits to the immune system, so taking a medicinal mushroom blend is a powerful choice. Many mushroom supplement companies have "immunity" blends that include all seven of the mushrooms mentioned in this book.

And some say, as with the "entourage effect" seen in cannabis, taking multiple mushrooms together can be more effective than taking just one. Read more on mushrooms and immunity in the cancer section.

How to use medicinal mushrooms to support the immune system:

- **Add a blend of medicinal mushrooms to your daily regimen.** Chaga, reishi, turkey tail, shiitake, maitake, lion's mane, and cordyceps have all been shown to have immune-balancing effects and antioxidants, which fight free radicals in the body. You can find blends in tincture or powder form to add to a daily smoothie or tea, and you can also find mushroom blends in capsules.

- **If you're coming down with a cold, take a chaga or reishi tincture (or drink chaga or reishi tea) every day.** Chaga and reishi are both powerhouses for immunity, and their potent medicinal properties can ward off sickness and boost you back to vitality.

- **Cook with medicinal mushrooms, especially shiitake and maitake.** Lentinan, the active compound in shiitake mushrooms, has been widely studied for its immune system–enhancing effects. A compound in maitake mushrooms called D-fraction has been shown to support the immune system and fight cancer cells. To add an extra immune system boost to your daily life, add shiitake and maitake to your cooking wherever you'd normally use any culinary mushroom!

Other Rebel immunity tips:

- **Turmeric.** The active compound in turmeric root (curcumin) is one of the most potent anti-inflammatory and immune-boosting supplements out there. You can use the turmeric root powder in cooking, drink a turmeric tea, or take it as capsules. Add turmeric powder as a spice to soups, stews, eggs, veggies, or any savory dish.

- **Garlic.** Garlic is sometimes referred to as "nature's antibiotic," and it can play a role in keeping the immune system strong. Add garlic to your immune-boosting regimen by incorporating it generously into your cooking. You can even swallow a chopped-up clove of raw garlic whole if you're coming down with something—warning, though—you will have garlic breath!

- **Elderberry.** Elderberry is one of the favorites for the immune system among herbalists. It's high in antioxidants, can help fight colds and the flu, and can boost the immune system—and researchers have found that compounds from elderberries can strengthen the immune response to viruses. You can find elderberry syrup at most health-food stores or online, or even make your own at home.

- **Raw honey.** Raw honey, in addition to being a delicious way to sweeten your foods or beverages, has antibacterial, anti-inflammatory, and antioxidant properties. If you can find local raw honey, it can help combat seasonal allergies.

- **Ginger.** Ginger is known to be anti-inflammatory and antibacterial, and can soothe nausea and support healthy digestion. One of my favorite immune-support beverages is ginger tea with a touch of raw honey, a squeeze of lemon juice, and a small pinch of cayenne pepper.

- **Sleep.** Getting enough sleep is the ultimate foundation for a healthy immune system. During sleep, our body is detoxifying, repairing, healing, and restoring. Sleep deprivation has been shown to elevate stress levels and increase inflammation, so prioritize your rest to accelerate your body's natural healing response.

Terpene Tip: Caryophyllene is the only terpene that also acts as a cannabinoid—and as there are cannabinoid receptors located throughout the immune system, cannabis varieties high in caryophyllene can help to modulate and balance immune system activity.

Rebel Ritual: Add a teaspoon of medicinal mushrooms and a dropperful of full-spectrum CBD oil to any smoothie for daily immune support.

SUPERFOOD OATMEAL

CONTRIBUTED BY DR. JEREMY GOLDBERG

My friend Dr. Jeremy Goldberg of Long Distance Love Bombs makes superfood oatmeal most mornings, and he always uses a different variety of superfood ingredients. Jeremy calls this his "Ninja-Proof Oatmeal Concoction." You can mix up or swap the ingredients however you like—the point is, you're majorly upgrading your everyday oatmeal!

Makes 1–2 servings

Oatmeal:

½–1 cup organic oats (Jeremy prefers the quick oats.)

1–2 cups of water (2 cups of water for every 1 cup of oatmeal, or follow package directions)

Superfood Suggestions (mix and match)

1 tsp. or more of the following:

Cacao

Coconut oil or MCT oil (you can use your CBD-infused coconut oil here!)

Nut butter (peanut, almond, or cashew)

Chia seeds

Goji berries

Mushroom powder of choice (chaga, reishi, lion's mane, or cordyceps are great choices here)

Maca

Spirulina, moringa, or greens powder

Flaxseeds

Top with:

A dash of cinnamon

A few drops of your favorite CBD oil

First, make your oatmeal as you normally would with oats and hot water, as directed on the package of oats you choose.

In a bowl you love that makes your heart sing, add your oatmeal and top with all of your superfoods.

Gently stir your superfoods into the oatmeal.

Add a dash of cinnamon on top.

Drizzle with a few drops of CBD oil.

Other variations to try: top with your favorite fruits (a kiwi, sliced strawberries, blueberries, blackberries, banana slices) or nuts (pistachios, walnuts, cashews, brazil).

CASHEW CHAGA LATTE

CONTRIBUTED BY HEALTH COACH AMANDA CARNEY

Amanda Carney is one of the best health coaches I know. A few years ago, we lived in apartments across the hall from each other in Brooklyn (yes, just like in *Friends*!), and we were both working as health coaches in Dr. Frank Lipman's functional medicine practice. I would often knock on her door in the morning so we could have coffee together. She'd always be whipping up some sort of delicious healthy latte and was happily willing to share. Now I'm paying it forward by sharing her immune-supporting chaga latte with you!

Makes 1 serving

1 cup brewed (organic) coffee (or herbal tea, if you are avoiding caffeine)

1 Tbsp. organic raw cashew butter

1 tsp. chaga mushroom powder (or whichever mushroom you're working with)

½ cup hot water

1 tsp. pure maple syrup (optional, for sweetness)

Place all ingredients in a blender and blend for 5–10 seconds, until frothy. Pour into your favorite mug and enjoy.

SOME OPTIONAL ADDITIONS INCLUDE:

½ tsp. reishi

½ dropperful of mushroom tincture

½ dropperful of CBD oil (your preferred dose)

Pinch of ashwagandha (start small—this is a bitter herb)

1 Tbsp. collagen powder

Sprinkle of cinnamon

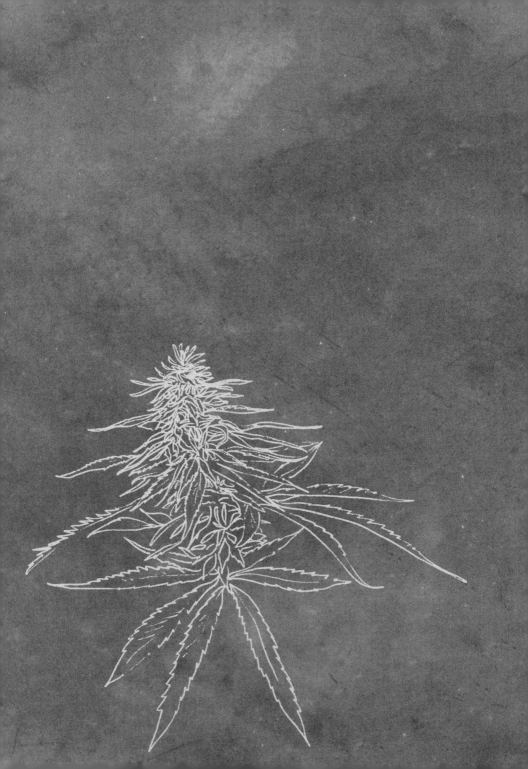

SUPERCHARGE YOUR SEX DRIVE

When you're stressed, anxious, tired, or sick, your libido can drop to the point where it feels nonexistent. Your sex drive is highly connected to your creative energy and overall vitality—in fact, some consider sexual energy to be the ultimate creative energy—it's the energy that creates life, after all. While getting enough sleep, lowering your level of stress, exercising (get those endorphins!), and feeling healthy and vibrant in general may be the best way to enhance your overall libido, cannabis and mushrooms can both help to supercharge your sex drive (and, therefore, your creative energy) when you need a little boost.

CBD can help you relax, unwind, and release anxiety—which is a huge step in the right direction when it comes to feeling sexy and sensual. In addition, small doses of THC can enhance your sensory experience—touch can feel more stimulating, music is more enjoyable, and taste is elevated. Many people report heightened physical sensation and pleasure when they consume a little bit of THC, and there are even CBD and THC personal lubricant products available, which, according to dispensary employees, are very popular.

Be cautious when using THC to enhance your sex drive, as taking too much THC can have the opposite effect than you want—leaving you feeling anxious, paranoid, or tired (this isn't typically the case with THC topicals or personal lubricants, though, so feel free to go wild with those).

A few ways to use cannabis to enhance your libido:

- Consume CBD as you normally would for anxiety (for instance, a tincture or herbal vaporizer) for a quick dose of relaxation and to take the edge off.

- Use a tiny dose of THC (start with 1–2 mg) for sensory enhancement.

- Use a CBD or THC massage oil with your partner (or on your own).

- Try a CBD or THC personal lubricant.

Of all the mushrooms in *The Rebel's Apothecary*, cordyceps is the one best known for being an aphrodisiac. It stimulates oxygen flow, blood flow, and energy throughout the body, which can heighten libido and enhance physical stamina. Cordyceps has also been shown to boost testosterone and improve sperm quality and hormonal balance (potentially improving fertility), and it has been known to increase libido in both sexes. A 2016 paper published in *Austin Andrology* even called cordyceps "a natural Himalayan Viagra."

How to use mushrooms to enhance your libido:

- Cordyceps can be added to your daily routine as a capsule, tincture, or powder extract. Take the recommended dose on the package of the product you choose and try it for a week or two to see what effects you notice.

- Add a teaspoon of cordyceps powder to hot water and drink it as a tea, or add it to your daily coffee.

- Add a teaspoon of cordyceps powder to a smoothie (such as The Ultimate Aphrodisiac Smoothie recipe, coming up next).

MAGIC MUSHROOM NOTE: Many people report heightened sensory enhancement and a libido boost after taking microdoses of psilocybin mushrooms—not enough to feel psychedelic effects, but just enough to feel that your sensory experience is slightly enhanced. (Again, these mushrooms are currently illegal, and it is not recommended to use them without the guidance of a trained psychedelic therapist.)

THE ULTIMATE APHRODISIAC SMOOTHIE

If you really want to start your day feeling turned on and full of sensual, creative energy, try this energizing aphrodisiac smoothie. Don't say I didn't warn you, though—this smoothie is a very *potent* aphrodisiac! Drink it and you'll be buzzing all day.

Makes 2 servings

1 dropperful of full-spectrum CBD oil (you choose your desired dose)

1 tsp. cordyceps mushroom powder

2–3 fresh or dried figs (depending on the level of sweetness you like)

1 Tbsp. cacao powder

2 tsp. maca powder

1 cup unsweetened coconut or almond milk

1 cup water (or another cup of milk if you want it to be creamier)

Tiny pinch of cayenne

Tiny pinch of ginger (powdered or fresh)

1 tsp. cinnamon

¼ avocado

½ tsp. vanilla extract

A touch of raw honey for sweetness (optional)

Add all ingredients to a blender, blend, and sip.

CREAMY DREAMY CBD HONEY CUPS

CONTRIBUTED BY KENDRA ADACHI

Chocolate, cannabis, rose petals, and honey? I can't think of a more sensual combination. Cannabis and cacao are a truly beautiful pair, and these creamy, dreamy honey cups are the perfect way to treat yourself or someone you love. Kendra Adachi is a plant-focused chef and health and mindset coach, who frequently infuses CBD into her recipes. You will need cupcake liners and a muffin tin for this recipe.

Makes 6 honey cups in a regular muffin tin or 12 small cups in a mini muffin tin

Chocolate Coating:

  1 dropperful of CBD oil (choose your desired dose)

  ¾ cup coconut oil, melted

  4–5 Tbsp. raw cacao powder (depending on how rich and dark you desire), plus more to taste

  ½ tsp. Himalayan salt or to taste

  1–2 Tbsp. pure maple syrup or alternative sweetener (use 5 drops liquid stevia for reduced sugar) or to taste

Creamy Dreamy Filling:

  ½ cup runny, smooth tahini

  1 dropperful CBD oil

  ¼ tsp. Himalayan salt

  ⅛–¼ cup runny honey (buckwheat honey is amazing in this recipe)

Garnish Ideas (optional):

Dried rose petals

Crushed pistachios

Himalayan salt

DIRECTIONS FOR CHOCOLATE COATING:

Mix the CBD oil with melted coconut oil and stir to combine.

Add cacao powder and mix until there are no clumps. Taste and add more cacao if desired.

Mix in salt and sweetener of choice, adjusting according to taste.

Put cupcake liners in a muffin tin and spoon approximately 1 tsp. (or ½ tsp. for 12 mini cups) chocolate coating into the bottom of each liner. The additional chocolate you have left will be used to top the creamy dreamy filling.

Place tin with liners in freezer to set, and keep remaining chocolate coating at room temperature while preparing the filling.

DIRECTIONS FOR CREAMY DREAMY FILLING:

In a bowl, combine the tahini, CBD oil, and salt. Mix thoroughly.

Swirl in the honey, not combining completely, leaving pockets of sweet surprises in the filling.

Remove chocolate from the freezer. Spoon 1 Tbsp. (or ½ tsp. for 12 mini cups) of the creamy dreamy filling into each cup, covering the chocolate base—being sure that each cup gets a swirl of honey with the mixture.

Cover the filling with remaining chocolate coating.

Optional: Add a pinch of each garnish: dried rose petals, crushed pistachios, and salt.

Place back in the freezer to set for 30 minutes. Enjoy! Store in freezer for 2–3 months.

Other ideas and recommendations: In place of tahini, experiment with roasted almond butter and mesquite, or cashew butter and maca.

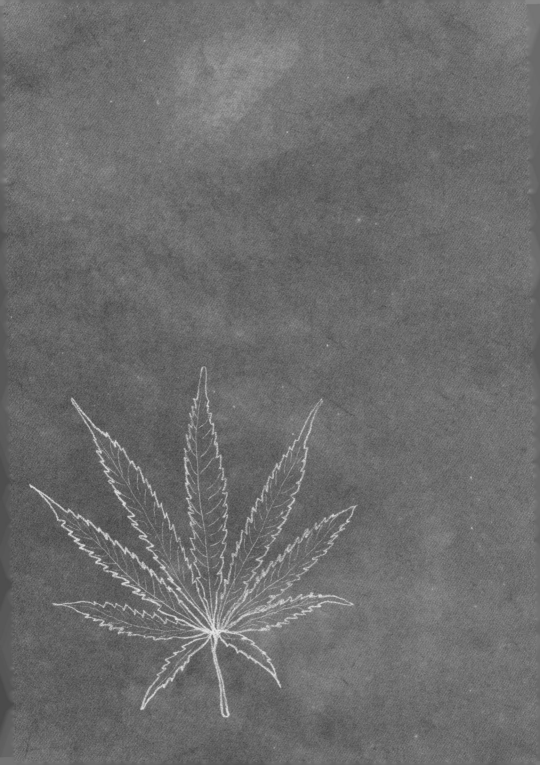

NOURISH YOUR SKIN

Our skin is the body's largest organ—and it just happens to be covered with cannabinoid receptors! We have both CB1 and CB2 receptors in our skin cells, and using cannabis topically can provide a host of benefits for the skin. According to a 2019 paper in the *Journal of Dermatological Treatment,* using cannabinoids topically has been shown to help with skin conditions such as acne, psoriasis, eczema, and even skin cancer. It's no wonder that skincare enthusiasts are raving about the benefits of cannabis products for clear skin and a radiant complexion. Because CBD and THC are both anti-inflammatory, topicals can be extremely soothing to irritated skin. Our body's own endocannabinoid system regulates inflammation in the skin and produces anti-inflammatory effects as needed—and using cannabis topically can enhance and support the endocannabinoid system.

How to use cannabis for skincare:

- Use a lotion, oil, or topical on your body that includes soothing CBD.

- Add a few drops of your CBD tincture to your daily face cream.

- Use a cannabis-infused face or body oil with both CBD and THC—these can be found at many dispensaries.

- Take cannabis tinctures internally—cannabinoids are anti-inflammatory and soothing to the whole system. What we take internally affects our skin.

CANNABIS-INFUSED "FACE MAGIC" OIL

CONTRIBUTED BY JANNA AND CHAD HOCKENJOS

Janna Hockenjos (one of my lovely, all-star book editors!) and her husband, Chad, use a cannabis-infused face oil every night. They love the skin-soothing effects of this oil so much, they even make it as gifts for friends!

Just as you would any moisturizer, this can be the next step after you cleanse and dry your face. As a bonus, you can customize it based on your skincare needs by adding a few drops of an essential oil.

Not only is this oil good for your skin, but if you take some time to massage it into the muscles of your jaw, cheeks, forehead, and anywhere you might feel tension, that tension will melt away.

Makes 4 oz.

⅔ cup cannabis-infused coconut oil (page 140; alternatively, ⅔ cup coconut oil plus 2 dropperfuls of your favorite unflavored CBD oil)

A few drops of the essential oil of your choice:

For oily skin: ylang-ylang oil

For dry skin: lemon + lavender oils

For acne: helichrysum oil

For antiaging, wrinkle reduction, and repair: frankincense oil

In a bowl, combine all ingredients and whisk until well combined. If your coconut oil is solid, gently warm before mixing with other oils.

Add oil to a 4-oz. mason jar.

Keep oil in a cool, dry place.

To apply, after cleansing and drying your skin, use a dab of oil (about the size of dime) and smooth all over your face.

USING MUSHROOMS FOR SKINCARE

Medicinal mushrooms can also be powerhouses when it comes to skincare, as they're packed with antioxidants—which is why they're being added to beauty products like face and body lotions, serums, and face masks. Chaga and reishi are both highly anti-inflammatory, and when added to skincare products they can be extremely soothing to the skin, can reduce redness, and have been shown to help with skin issues such as rosacea, eczema, and psoriasis. Shiitake has been known to fight hyperpigmentation and can help clear up sun spots. Tremella is another skin-loving mushroom to be on the lookout for in your beauty products, as it's hyper-moisturizing. As all of the medicinal mushrooms are rich in antioxidants and highly anti-inflammatory, they can be a worthy addition to your skincare routine.

Beauty products aside, mushrooms taken internally can also help the skin—so don't skimp on taking those double-extracted mushroom tinctures!

How to Get Started with Mushrooms for Skincare:

- Take chaga, shiitake, or reishi internally in a powder, tincture, or in tea or food. What you put into your body has a major effect on the way your skin looks and feels, as the skin is one of our largest organs of elimination.

- You can either use skincare products that have medicinal mushrooms added to them, or add a little bit of your own mushroom tincture or powder to your favorite lotion, cream, or face mask.

MUSHROOM FACE MASK

Here's a recipe for a homemade face mask with powdered medicinal mushrooms, moisturizing avocado, and raw honey, which is antibacterial:

1 Tbsp. raw honey

¼ avocado

1 tsp. mushroom powder (try chaga or reishi)

Mix ingredients together in a bowl until well combined. Apply to clean, freshly washed and dried face with your fingertips. Leave on for 15–30 minutes and wash off.

MORNING-TO-EVENING REBEL RITUALS

Morning: Enhance energy and focus, calm anxiety

Afternoon: General wellness, energy boosting,
immune-system support

Evening: Relaxation, stress relief, and sleep

ere are a few examples of how you can add some of the rebel rituals in this book into your daily life. These are just suggestions, so get creative and turn your own home into a Rebel's Apothecary that's unique to you!

Morning

- Take a low dose of a CBD tincture for focus and anxiety relief (try 5–10 mg to start)

- Add lion's mane extract to your morning beverage for brain power, or try the Focus Elixir (page 213)

- Boost a smoothie with a mushroom blend or low dose of CBD—try the Rebel's Green Smoothie (page 164)

- Mix cordyceps into your tea or coffee for sustained energy— try the Morning Adaptogenic Elixir (page 217)

- Cook a mushroom-rich breakfast with sautéed shiitakes, eggs, and arugula, or make Superfood Oatmeal (page 226)

Afternoon

- Drink a mug of chaga tea for immune system support—or try the Cashew Chaga Latte (page 228)

- Make a matcha tea with added lion's mane extract for a steady stream of focused energy—try the Adaptogenic Matcha Cold Brew (page 215)

- Add CBD Tahini Dressing (page 151) or CBD Pesto (page 60) to your lunch

- Sprinkle the Shiitake or Maitake Bacon (page 154) on a salad

- Take a low dose of CBD for anxiety relief and focus (try 5–10 mg to start)

- Try an energy-boosting snack: Cordyceps Energy Bars (page 219) , Healthy CBD Gummies (page 201), or Rebel's Green Juice (page 218)

Evening

- Add medicinal mushrooms into your cooking—try the Shiitake Mushroom Broth (page 158), Grilled Maitake Mushrooms (page 161), or Lion's Mane Braised in Coconut (page 157)

- Lather on a soothing CBD- or THC-rich massage oil to help you relax

- Use a 1:1 CBD-to-THC transdermal compound for any areas of pain before bedtime

- Take a higher dose of a CBD tincture at night for deep relaxation, with a little bit of THC if you tolerate it well (try 25 mg of CBD—or more, if needed)

- Sip a calming mug of reishi tea or the Starlight Tonic (page 176) for grounding and stress relief

- Enjoy Freezer Fudge "Pot Brownies," (page 187), Sautéed Peaches and Figs with Canna-Coconut Oil (page 148), or Creamy Dreamy CBD Honey Cups (page 235) for dessert

Nature itself is the best physician.

—*Hippocrates*

PART 3
NEXT-LEVEL REBELS

Therapeutic Doses and Advanced Cases

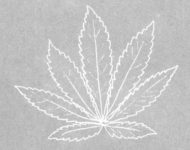

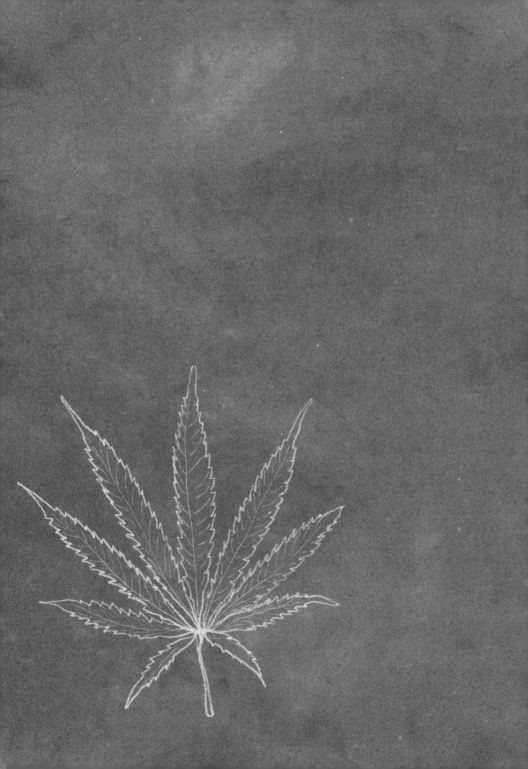

USING CANNABIS AND MUSHROOMS DURING CANCER TREATMENT

A NOTE FROM MY DAD

don't know how you prepare for it. It's scary. Pancreatic cancer especially—I knew a few people who had it, and they passed away quickly. Everything you read about, along with some of the things the doctors told me early on—there wasn't really any good news in it. The numbers around pancreatic cancer are undeniably dismal. My tumor couldn't be surgically removed because it had spread to the liver, so from what I understood, the goal of treatment is to live as normally as you can, for as long as you can. That's fairly sobering news. Everybody knows that life goes on for only so long, but I don't know how you prepare for a diagnosis like that. "You have pancreatic cancer, it's stage four, and it's very unlikely that anything other than a predictable road to your demise is what's coming next." That's what my story was.

The things that came to my mind first were all that I was going to miss—the things I had been looking forward to. This is probably true for everyone who's faced with a serious health problem. *This good life is going to be shorter than I had hoped,* I thought. I was going to miss Ashley's wedding, and how *Game of Thrones* ended. I was going to miss going to Myrtle Beach and playing golf with my high school friends.

My diagnosis came right before Thanksgiving, and the golf trip was planned for April. When I asked my doctor whether or not I'd make it to that golf trip, although his attitude was positive, he was noncommittal. So that felt really sad. As selfish as it sounds, I was worried that all the fun I had planned might not come true.

As I write this, it's been more than two years since my diagnosis—and my story has changed. I feel great. I'm on vacation with my family, I've played golf several times this week . . . and I did get to see the end of *Game of Thrones!*

In the spring, I told my oncologist that I was out in the yard doing some cleanup after a bad winter. He shook his head and said, "Most people in your condition are lying on the couch watching old movies at this point." I said, "I have plenty of energy, I have plenty of strength, and I feel good. So, I'm cutting up tree branches, doing yard work, and enjoying myself."

My oncologist sees a lot of very sick people and has a lot of hard conversations. But in my meetings, there's a lot of laughing. We have the same conversation every time. "Blood work is good, scans are terrific, you're off the charts in terms of how well you're doing. How's your golf game?"

Early on, some of the questions the doctors and nurses asked me were: "Are you falling down? Do you have bad nausea? Are you dropping things yet? Can you still type?" and I thought, *Uh oh—those are the things that are coming next.* But they haven't. Early on, I had a couple of bouts of nausea, but nothing like what you read about—no debilitating nausea at all.

I'm aware that my progress is atypical, being this deep into the disease that I have. Still, it doesn't appear to be getting worse . . . and it might actually be getting better.

I'm conservative, generally a believer in science and Western medicine—always have been. The first thing that came to my mind when I got diagnosed was, *I have cancer, I have to find the best cancer hospital that I can.* My daughter Lisa helped me get an appointment at Dana Farber in Boston. It never even crossed my mind to think about alternative medicine. I was going to do whatever conventional Western medicine told me to do—that just made sense to me.

Until I saw a documentary about medical marijuana. I only recorded it because it looked interesting. Ever since the 1960s, when marijuana was common in college, I thought of it as an illegal recreational drug. I didn't think it was dangerous, and I didn't believe it was the worst thing you could do—but I certainly didn't think of it as a medicine.

Yet here I was, watching a documentary where children having seizures were being given cannabis oil, after all conventional medicines they tried had been ineffective. The seizures immediately seemed to get better. You watch this and you say, "Okay, something's here. I don't know what it is, but this is pretty interesting."

I researched a little further and found anecdotal story after story, and it appeared that this stuff has some medicinal power. I started to change my viewpoint. I started to think, *Well, I'm going to go down the conventional medicine pathway, but if my oncologist says cannabis might do some good and it won't do any harm, why not try it?*

I trusted my daughter Jenny to guide me in creating a home regimen because she has as much history in researching these kinds of things as anybody I know. She's studied nutrition and she's an advocate for everything she believes might help people to feel healthier and live a better life. This seemed to be an extension of what she was already involved in.

Ever since Jenny has been studying nutrition, she's spent a lot of time and energy trying to teach me about it—but I'm an old dog, and I don't like too many new tricks. But this time, I thought—*Maybe it's time to learn a new trick.*

When you're sick, time is important. We decided in the course of just one day to get a medical marijuana card, get some CBD and medicinal mushrooms, and get started.

It's hard to say what's direct cause and effect, but it's also hard for me to ignore the fact that I'm still as healthy as before I was diagnosed, and maybe healthier. Western medicine predicted that I'd be in *much* worse condition than I am.

Two years into chemo, I still have no nausea, and I have a lot fewer "old-man pains" than I used to have. I used to take over-the-counter pain medications every day for joint pain, but I don't take those things anymore. After starting CBD oil, I just don't have the same pain as I used to have. Something's working.

Before now, the only mushrooms I had ever heard about in terms of medicines were—well, I don't think I had heard of any, except things that were way on the fringes, like psilocybin. Medicinal mushrooms were nowhere near my field of view, so bringing them in was purely faith that they aren't going to hurt me and that they might do some good.

In the two years since we've started this, it feels like the world has changed quite a bit. There's certainly an increasing amount of evidence that cannabis and mushrooms can have a major impact on certain health issues, and it's highly probable that this is not just a placebo effect.

I've since learned that the cannabis plant has been used as a medicine around the world for thousands of years. One hundred years ago, marijuana was demonized, even though there's almost no evidence that there's anything in it that's bad for you. They turned it into a reefer-madness issue, which is still a big part of society. I don't believe in that anymore. This is not something that's going to do more harm than the potential good it can do. The evidence is mounting on a daily basis that it can be beneficial, so the idea that we're still prohibiting it, to me, is wacky. But reefer madness has been so embedded in people's brains, it's hard to undo. But we can undo it, and it's being undone now.

I'm committed to this. I believe it's helping to keep me healthy, giving me a good quality of life, and extending my life a lot longer than the doctors would have thought.

When you go to the doctor and they say, "We can keep you alive for a while, but it won't be all that pleasant. You're going to have neuropathy and nausea, you're going to be weak and tired and sick"—that's when I think it's time to add on to conventional medicine. I'm not going against conventional medicine, but I'm now much more open to trying alternatives. I think someday, these "alternatives" won't be all that unconventional.

The more I hear about patients with cancer, I can see that it becomes a real emotional drain—a helplessness. I don't feel that way. Of course, you feel like you're at the mercy of your cancer hospital in some respects, but I don't feel emotionally down, because the idea that I could try something at home to support my treatment and have it work, well, that's great. It's invigorating. I get up, I feel good, I continue to mark off the months on the calendar, and nothing is going wrong. It's emotionally uplifting. I don't get depressed very often. Of course, I wish I wasn't on this path—but it's still been a pretty interesting and positive experience. It's actually been kind of fun to try all of this, and to see it working. If it wasn't working, it wouldn't be any fun at all, but since it is, I'm going to continue to do it.

If what I'm sharing can help other people, and possibly accelerate the acceptance of cannabis and mushrooms by people in the medical community, if I'm just one voice in an increasing number of voices that say, "Hey, you might want to look into this," and help people see that maybe it doesn't have to be a quick death sentence, if this gives the medical community another data point—well, all the better. The faster we can get to clinical trials, the better off a lot of people are going to be. So how could I not share this?

Today, it's not only "So far, so good." It's "So far, *unbelievably* good." There are so few positive outcomes with this disease that my oncologist told us to share every positive thing about this story that we possibly can. This has been a very pleasant surprise, and I believe that we caused it—at least some of it—by taking some action at home, in conjunction with conventional medicine.

This might sound crazy, but this has been one of the best times of my life. The specifics of getting chemotherapy aren't pleasant, but the last two years have been phenomenally fun. I'm spending much more time with my family and friends. Every day, week, month (and now, every year) ends up being a gift. I'm not just lying on the couch watching movies.

If I didn't know I was sick, I wouldn't know I was sick—and I'm having the time of my life. It's just the truth.

What I wish for you, the reader of this book, if you're open-minded enough to try what I'm trying, is that you get up and take some action. My experience is my experience, but trying cannabis and mushrooms probably won't hurt, it could do some good, and it could improve your probabilities. There's a lot of hope that you can feel better than your doctors think you can—better than *you* think you can.

If there's one thing I can say for sure, it's this:

Even if the probabilities aren't great, the *possibilities* are great.

Ray Sansouci

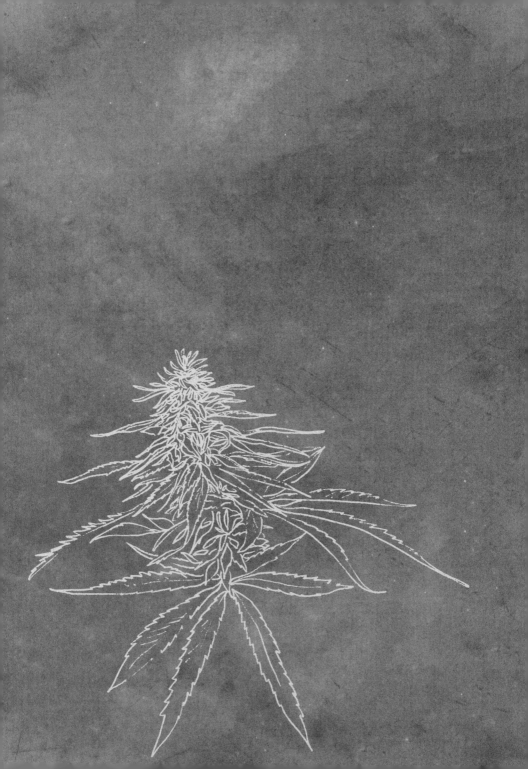

USING ALTERNATIVE THERAPIES
AND TALKING TO YOUR DOCTOR

I f you've been through the life-changing moment when you hear that you or someone you love has cancer, you are far from alone. In 2018, an estimated 17 million people worldwide were diagnosed with cancer—and that diagnosis affects many more people than just the cancer patient.

When I first searched "pancreatic cancer," it was difficult to find any positive information. Now my hope is that I can help change that. The most fulfilling emails I've ever received have been the ones from newly diagnosed patients and caregivers, saying that my blogs on cancer were the only thing they could find on the Internet that has given them hope and inspiration in a sea of not-so-positive information. Just hearing that someone else has been able to enjoy life and feel good during cancer treatment can be a tremendous relief.

When I told my dad's oncologist that I planned to write about this topic, he said, "Spread as much positive information as you can about this disease. People need to know that it's not all doom and gloom."

If you or someone you love recently got a cancer diagnosis, there's no way around the fact that it feels scary and disorienting. After the initial disbelief from getting a cancer diagnosis starts to settle, there can be a feeling of hopelessness that sets in. But the situation doesn't have to be hopeless, and conventional treatments aren't the *only* option for supporting your health and healing. There are ways that you can feel good and healthy and have a great quality of life, even during conventional cancer treatments. You have the power to enhance how good you can feel during treatment—and potentially, possibly . . . help fight the cancer, too. The goal of *The Rebel's Apothecary* is to help you feel as healthy and supported as possible along the way.

More research is happening every day that focuses on the addition of cannabis and medicinal mushrooms as adjunct cancer therapies— both to alleviate side effects of conventional treatments and to potentially kill cancer cells, too. In fact, there's been evidence that cannabis and medicinal mushrooms can actually help conventional cancer treatments such as chemotherapy work *better*. By the time this book lands in your hands, there will likely be even more research to support this.

In case I haven't said it enough, creating your own Rebel's Apothecary isn't about denying conventional cancer treatments or going against your doctor's recommendations. It's about giving yourself the greatest amount of support possible for your health and healing. I can't tell you what the best option is for you when it comes to treating your cancer, of course, but whatever you choose to do, please know that you have some wonderful natural options that can complement your doctor's plan for you, support you through the process, relieve you of some of the negative side effects of your treatment, and majorly improve your quality of life.

TALK TO YOUR ONCOLOGIST

First and foremost, please know that much of the information I'm sharing in this book hasn't been verified through clinical trials yet. The information I'm presenting here is in no way intended to replace your doctor's advice, nor should it be considered a medical recommendation. My intention is that this book points you in a direction of information gathering and experimenting for yourself, in the way that feels right for you, your family, and your doctor.

If you decide to support your cancer treatments with cannabis, medicinal mushrooms, or any other herb or supplement, talk to your oncologist about it first. Create a plan that everyone is on board with, and when you first have the conversation with your doctor, go into the meeting prepared with your own proposed ideas, research, and information. Don't expect your oncologist to know enough about cannabis and mushrooms to be able to give you a fully informed opinion. These remedies likely weren't a part of your doctor's training (although this is changing!), and they may not have any experience with these remedies. I suspect that as legality shifts and more clinical research is done, oncologists will be required to know how to speak to their patients about medical cannabis and medicinal mushrooms—but for now, your doctor might tell you they simply don't know enough about it to recommend it.

When my dad first started chemo, we told his oncologist that he was going to experiment with medical cannabis, and we brought in some of the medicinal mushroom supplements we were thinking about trying. His doctor suggested to tread carefully with these remedies because he didn't have any clinical evidence that they would help, but he also said that "it probably won't hurt." We accepted that as a green light. My dad's progress would be monitored every two weeks at the cancer hospital, so we knew we would have frequent check-ins about not only the tumors but about his quality of life and any side effects. We could stop using cannabis or mushrooms anytime if he had any kind of negative reaction to them. For us, the positive anecdotal evidence and preliminary research were enough for us to believe they were worth a try.

WHAT TO DO IF YOUR DOCTOR SAYS "NO"

American oncologists commonly tell patients to
avoid all dietary supplements and natural remedies while
undergoing treatment, and to eat whatever they want.
That's not good enough. I would urge patients and families
not to reject surgery, chemotherapy, or radiotherapy,
but to seek and demand integrative treatment.

—*Dr. Andrew Weil*

When I first started sharing about this cancer journey online, I got emails from patients and caregivers saying their doctor "won't allow" them to use medical cannabis, CBD, or medicinal mushrooms, despite the positive stories and research about people boosting their immune systems, alleviating their chemotherapy side effects, and helping them fight the cancer. The people who get in touch with me are often in pain, losing too much weight, and their immune systems are breaking down. They are often desperate for a solution, and some of these natural remedies *may* help. In some cases, they may help a lot.

Instead of asking your doctor for "permission" to try these remedies, it might be a more fruitful conversation to ask if there are any *specific* concerns your doctor has about them related to you or the medications you're taking. If your doctor says a firm "no" to you about adding cannabis or medicinal mushrooms to your cancer treatment plan, make sure you dig into their reasoning a little bit more before accepting it as truth.

Questions to ask your doctor:

- Are they saying no because of a specific reason that's unique to you, your condition, or your medications?

- Is there research they are basing their answer on?

- What is the specific drawback they are concerned about?

- Is it because the doctor doesn't have enough experience with cannabis and mushrooms to officially recommend them?

- If that's the case, would they be willing to get on board with you trying any of these remedies for just one scan cycle, and then reassessing as a team?

Of course, cannabis and mushrooms may not be right for you. Every case is different, every person is different, and every cancer is different.

If your doctor says there will be a drug interaction with a medication you're already taking, or that there's evidence to support the fact that these remedies will be harmful to you, of course you want to take that seriously—but make sure to ask them for the information they're looking at in order to come to that conclusion.

It's your body and your health we're talking about, so it's important to understand why you're taking—or not allowed to take—any drug, plant, or supplement. If you don't understand, keep asking questions until you do.

Don't be afraid to get a second opinion, or a third opinion. If you share your doctor's viewpoint, that's great. The mind is powerful, and believing in your treatment is important.

STAY CURIOUS. KEEP ASKING QUESTIONS. THIS IS YOUR HEALTH, YOUR BODY, AND YOUR *LIFE*.

NOW THAT YOU'RE READY . . .

If you've come to the conclusion that you're ready to experiment with medical cannabis or medicinal mushrooms to support your cancer treatment, and you've gotten your oncologist on board, too, in the next section you'll find tips on how to get started.

CANNABIS AND CANCER

The National Cancer Institute has noted on its website that "cannabis has been shown to kill cancer cells in the laboratory" and that cannabinoids appear to kill tumor cells while leaving non-cancer cells intact—which is the primary goal of any cancer treatment. The National Institute on Drug Abuse says on their website, "Marijuana extracts may help kill certain cancer cells and reduce the size of others."

A recent study on pancreatic cancer in mice showed that the addition of cannabis inhibited tumor growth, significantly improved survival rates, and seemed to boost the effectiveness of chemotherapy drugs.

If larger-scale studies can be done showing these results, cannabis could become a frontline treatment for cancer. For now, cannabis doctors often recommend that cancer patients focus on getting as many cannabinoids into the body as possible, with dosage dependent on THC tolerance.

At the time of this writing, thirty-three states in the United States have medical cannabis programs. Federal legalization is expected within the coming years, so with that shift, I hope all cancer patients who want to use cannabis will have access to it easily and affordably.

RICK SIMPSON OIL, OR RSO

We can't talk about cannabis and cancer without mentioning Rick Simpson Oil. When I get emails from people who have been newly diagnosed with cancer, one of the first questions they usually ask me is "Do you know anything about Rick Simpson Oil?" And I immediately smile, because I know this means they're on the right track. This oil is one of the most potent medical cannabis products available today, and it allows patients to administer a high dose of cannabinoids into the body quickly. It can be incredibly helpful for chemotherapy side effects—it can relieve nausea, increase appetite, elevate mood, and help with sleep.

Walk into any medical dispensary and the budtenders will know what you're talking about if you mention Rick Simpson Oil, or RSO. This oil gets its name from—you guessed it—a man named Rick Simpson, who used a high-potency homemade cannabis oil extract to treat and cure his own skin cancer. In cannabis oil, he found something that was effective, had a high safety profile, and had minimal side effects. He made it his mission to help other cancer patients with this oil, always making it for them at no cost.

Rick Simpson was one of the inspirations for the medical cannabis oil that many cancer patients are using today, and he's had to go through quite a bit of struggle and conflict with the legal and medical systems in order to help patients get access to this medicine.

I'm grateful that he kept fighting for this cause, because his work ultimately helped my dad and me to find the cannabis oil that he benefits from every day. My dad and I both believe it's this cannabis oil that has had the greatest effect on how well he's doing with his cancer treatments, and how high his quality of life has continued to be for the past two years. I believe that a Rick Simpson type of oil could be one of the most important medical products of our time, and I hope we will see more developments and research done in the future to prove this clinically.

Although Rick Simpson helped to popularize this cannabis oil, it must be noted that he doesn't personally produce or sell the oil his name appears on in cannabis dispensaries. These days, most dispensaries refer to the oil as RSO. He has, however, written two books about his experience with cannabis oil and cancer. There's a documentary about his work that's also worth watching, called *Run from the Cure*.

RSO is a highly concentrated oil, made by extracting the resins from cannabis flower with a solvent (such as alcohol), boiling off the residual solvents, and leaving behind only the oily medicinal resin. When I say high-potency, I mean it—this oil could have over 50 mg of THC (or CBD, depending on what kind you're getting) in just one drop!

> This harmless nonaddictive natural medication can be used with great success, to cure or control cancer, MS, pain, diabetes, arthritis, asthma, infections, inflammations, blood pressure, depression, sleeping problems and just about any other medical issues that one can imagine. We have been criticized for calling this oil a cure-all, but what else could you call a substance that can be used successfully to treat so many medical problems?
>
> —*Rick Simpson*

You may see various kinds of RSO-type oils at medical cannabis dispensaries—some with high-THC levels, some with high CBD
levels, and some with a more or less equal mix (a 1:1 ratio of CBD to
THC). The original oil that Rick Simpson has historically produced
is a high-THC variety—but many patients have found great success
with a 1:1 ratio of CBD to THC in this type of oil. The one my dad is
taking is a 1:1 ratio, which gives him equal amounts of medicine from
both CBD and THC.

If you choose a 1:1 oil, the CBD will mitigate some of the intoxicating effects from the THC, and as you know, they will work together
to enhance each other's medicinal benefits. If feeling high is an absolute "no" for you, stick with a higher-CBD ratio of this oil, if you can
find it.

If you are heading to a medical dispensary for the first time and want
to get your hands on some of this liquid gold, ask your friendly budtender to show you what the options are for "something similar to Rick
Simpson Oil or RSO." Oftentimes, medical dispensaries will have an
online menu, so you can check to see if this oil is available before you
make the trip. It may be listed on the website under extracts, oils, or
edible products. Sometimes it has a name like Full Extract Cannabis
Oil (FECO) or whole-plant extract. If you're unsure, ask the person
working at the dispensary. If you meet with a cannabis doctor to get
your medical card, they may be able to direct you to a local dispensary
that has this type of oil.

The oil typically comes in a plastic syringe (with no needle in it), so
you can squeeze it out in small drops to take the medicine orally. At this
time, it is generally sold at medical dispensaries in 1-g syringes.

The oil is potent, thick, and greasy—most patients report that it's
unpleasant to put into your mouth by itself. My dad puts his daily dose

onto a small bit of peanut butter and swallows it. Rick Simpson suggests folding it into a piece of bread.

The Rick Simpson protocol is to take 60 g of this oil over a ninety-day period. This equals a little bit more than half a gram per day, which can get very pricey—but I expect costs to go down as legalization becomes more widespread and more products become available.

While all cancers (and all cancer patients) are different, some have experienced success by taking up to 1 g of the 1:1 cannabis oil per day (500 mg of CBD and 500 mg of THC). This is a very large dose, and something that you'd have to work up to slowly to reduce the potentially uncomfortable intoxicating effects from the THC. Some doctors say the dose doesn't need to be this high, however—and people have experienced extraordinary benefits at lower doses.

As noted in MacCallum and Russo's 2018 paper in the *European Journal of Medicine*:

High doses (up to 1000 mg (1g)/d), preferably of mixed phytocannabinoids (as in cannabis extracts), for up to 3 months may be required to eradicate some malignancies, but emphasis is required that this approach remains anecdotal . . . high doses of THC-containing preparations require slow titration over 2 weeks to induce tolerance.

If you choose to try this oil to complement your cancer treatment, daily intake is recommended to experience the greatest benefit. "Taking a steady amount of a whole-plant extract works better than taking sporadic doses," says Dr. David Meiri, a cannabis and cancer researcher in Israel.

The protocol suggests to take this oil two or three times per day, starting with a tiny drop the size of half a grain of rice in each dose, and to increase your dose as tolerated every few days. Most people will feel a high from this product, so start very slowly. The frequency of your doses will depend on your tolerance to the THC in the oil.

My dad goes through 1 g of this oil in about five days, which could be considered a low amount compared to the recommended protocol, but it's helped him to feel great, his cancer remains stable, and at the time of this writing, he's been able to tolerate more than fifty rounds of a strong chemotherapy regimen over two years. Over the course of his chemotherapy treatments, he's increased his nighttime dose bit by bit, as he's less concerned with feeling THC's effects at night. Every time I call him, I lovingly encourage him to continue experimenting with upping his dose, and he always assures me he's at the highest dose he feels comfortable taking.

With some experimentation (ideally, under the guidance of a cannabis doctor), find the "sweet spot" that works for you—the dose that gives you the relief you want and helps you to experience positive progress on your cancer journey, but doesn't make you feel uncomfortable. This chapter should be enough to help you get started, and from here, your cannabis doctor and medical dispensary budtenders can lead you to the next steps.

For more on this oil and other experiences of cancer patients who have benefited from it, I highly suggest watching the documentary *Weed the People*, which follows the treatment of children with cancer using this specific type of high-potency cannabis oil.

The more time that goes by, the more I hear positive stories from other cancer patients taking this oil. I got an email the other day from a blog reader who said, "My sister is going through chemotherapy, and is now taking the cannabis oil every day. At first she was scared to feel

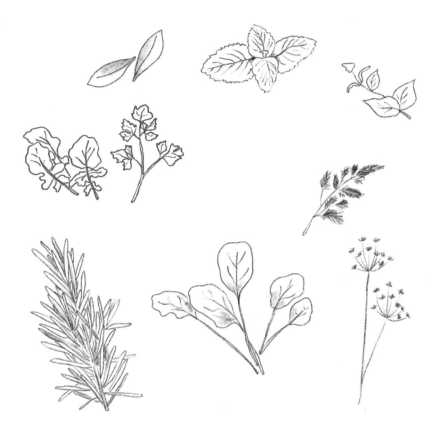

high, but you were right—she just had to work up very slowly. Now she's thrilled with the way it helps her sleep and increases her appetite. She's gaining weight back and feeling stronger every day."

Other Delivery Methods

If you can't find the specific oil I'm mentioning here, don't worry—just ask the budtender at the dispensary or a cannabis doctor to recommend an alternative. Tinctures and capsules are also great ways to get CBD and THC into your system, and if you can't find a 1:1 ratio, you can absolutely try another. The goal is to get cannabinoids into your system so the cannabis can start working its magic.

Using a variety of delivery methods for cannabis medicine is preferred during cancer treatment, to get systematic relief and receive a wide range of cannabinoids.

Many people find pain relief from certain types of cancer by using topicals or suppositories. These products can help to get as many cannabinoids as possible as close to the cancer as possible, so depending on where your cancer is located, these may be viable options for you.

Inhalation can be the quickest way to find relief from nausea and pain, and to stimulate appetite, so you may want to consider keeping some 1:1 CBD-to-THC flower and a dry herb vaporizer on hand for fast-acting relief.

In addition to physical health benefits, cannabis can help ease the depression and anxiety that may come with a cancer diagnosis. As cannabis journalist and author David Bienenstock writes in *Leafly,* "To laugh, to escape from pain and anxiety, to step outside one's self and experience a moment of peace, or bliss, or both—what could be more healing?"

IF YOU DON'T HAVE ACCESS TO MEDICAL CANNABIS

If you don't have access to medical cannabis but you do have access to CBD, I would start by getting a high-quality full-spectrum CBD oil that's been lab tested. A tincture or capsules would be a great place to start to get those cannabinoids into your body easily and efficiently. Some of the CBD oil brands I recommend at this time are in the Resources section of this book, and you can also head to

RebelsApothecary.com/Resources for updated information on CBD brands I use and recommend.

The Realm of Caring, a nonprofit that provides cannabis education to patients, recommends that adult cancer patients start at 50 mg of CBD two times daily (100 mg/day), and child cancer patients start at 25 mg of CBD two times daily (50 mg/day), and to move up with dosing as quickly as the individual can tolerate (many patients take up to 500 mg of CBD or more per day). Of course, work directly with a cannabis doctor, especially when dosing for children.

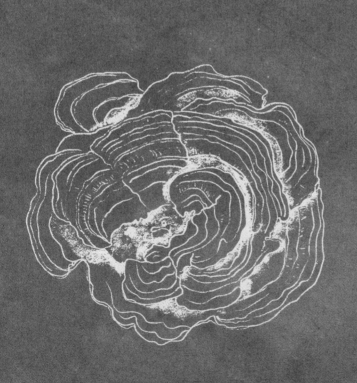

MEDICINAL MUSHROOMS AND CANCER

Medicinal mushrooms have been established as a novel and promising source for natural therapeutics that can be successfully applied in the treatment of different diseases, including cancer," says Professor Solomon P. Wasser.

Chaga, shiitake, turkey tail, maitake, cordyceps, lion's mane, and reishi all contain powerful beta-glucans that can be beneficial to support the immune system in fighting cancer and mitigate some of the side effects of chemotherapy. A good place to start with medicinal mushrooms (with your oncologist's approval) could be to try a blend of different medicinal mushrooms, in capsules, powder extracts, or tinctures.

Here are just a few examples of how mushrooms can potentially support cancer treatment:

- **Shiitake:** AHCC (activated hexose correlated compound), which is derived from shiitake mushrooms, has been shown in studies to be an immune system enhancer in people going through chemotherapy—it's used in over seven hundred hospitals in Japan.

The compound lentinan in shiitake has been shown to activate natural killer (NK) cells and increase white blood cells in the immune system.

- **Turkey tail:** Another superstar in the cancer field is turkey tail. In Japan, the main compound in turkey tail (Polysaccharide-K, or PSK) is an approved cancer drug called Krestin, and a Bastyr University study found that turkey tail mushrooms can stimulate the cancer-fighting response of the immune system in breast cancer patients.

- **Chaga:** Studies show the betulinic acid in wild-harvested chaga can slow tumor growth and induce apoptosis (cell death) in cancer cells. In Russia, a chaga extract called Befungin is an approved medicine for cancer patients.

- **Maitake:** D-fraction, the active polysaccharide in maitake mushrooms, has been widely studied for its antitumor activity and was approved as an adjunct therapeutic cancer drug in China in 2010.

- **Reishi:** The ganoderic acid in reishi has been shown to inhibit tumor growth, and it has been widely studied for its immune system modulating effects, in addition to being able to reverse resistance to chemotherapy drugs—potentially helping patients tolerate chemotherapy for a longer period of time.

- **Cordyceps:** In cordyceps, the active compound is called cordycepin, which has been shown to have antitumor and anti-metastatic properties, and can potentially help stop malignant cancer cells from spreading.

- **Lion's mane:** Last but not least, lion's mane—although this mushroom's superpowers lie primarily in cognitive function, the erinacines in lion's mane have also shown antitumor properties, particularly in the case of lung cancer.

"Mushroom extracts can lead to increased survival times and improved quality of life," says Dr. Christopher Hobbs, research scientist and author of *Medicinal Mushrooms.*

You can use medicinal mushroom blends if you want to take the whole arsenal of mushrooms at once, or you can pick and choose which mushrooms you want and take them separately. My dad drinks a smoothie every day with a powder blend of ten different medicinal mushrooms in it—that smoothie recipe is on page 289.

> **Rebel Ritual:** To bring more mushroom medicine into your daily life during cancer treatment, try using a variety of delivery methods. Take a potent mushroom tincture, a blend of medicinal mushrooms in a smoothie, and cook more with the culinary mushrooms whenever you can (shiitake, maitake, and lion's mane). Drink chaga and reishi in tea, as part of your evening routine.

Just as with cannabis, a variety of mushrooms in different forms could be the best way to support your whole body while going through cancer treatment. With mushrooms for immune support and cannabis to nourish the endocannabinoid system, you can create a well-rounded healing support regimen.

Psilocybin mushrooms (those are the psychedelic ones!) are currently being researched for potential therapeutic use for the depression and anxiety that often come with a cancer diagnosis. To stay up-to-date on this research and shifts in legality, head to RebelsApothecary.com /Resources.

Drug Interactions

Before you jump to add medicinal mushrooms, CBD, or any other herb or supplement to your healing plan, make sure to visit the Memorial Sloan Kettering Cancer Center (MSKCC) website at mskcc.org to see the list of potential drug interactions. Search "cannabis" or the specific name of the mushroom you're considering taking (for example, "chaga") in the search box at the top of the MSKCC site, and you will find a comprehensive, updated list of drug interactions there.

MANAGING CHEMOTHERAPY
SIDE EFFECTS

In the midst of winter, I found there was,

within me, an invincible summer.

—Albert Camus

My dad's oncologist recently told me that pancreatic cancer is likely only going to become more and more common, and will rise to be one of the leading causes of death within the next few years. "But what if we find a solution?" I asked him. He smiled. "Yes, well, that would be the ideal outcome, wouldn't it?"

Imagine a world where cannabis and medicinal mushrooms are used to treat cancer in hospitals everywhere. A world where all cannabis and mushroom products are not only known and understood but available to all patients. A world where patients don't have to suffer so greatly due to the side effects of conventional treatments, and there are fewer people getting cancer overall because the preventative effects of cannabis and medicinal mushrooms are so commonplace. Imagine that there are no longer any restraints on research and testing, and cancer isn't considered the dire diagnosis it is today.

When I spend time at the cancer hospital where my dad is being treated, I frequently imagine this world. I imagine the day when I hear the news—*We now have enough research on cannabis and mushrooms to conclude there is evidence beyond the shadow of a doubt that they help in the treatment of cancer and the management of symptoms.* On that day, I imagine cancer patients everywhere having their worlds opened up to new, affordable, accessible options they haven't had before. Where they can not only find information about cannabis and medicinal mushrooms in a book like this one but also hear it straight from their own doctor.

Conventional cancer treatments and pharmaceutical drugs are successfully treating all kinds of cancers and other diseases every day. There are incredible researchers and doctors in the oncology field that care deeply about their patients and are doing everything they possibly can to treat them in the best way possible.

I support the use of conventional medicine where it's useful, and I support advances in pharmaceutical research. However, a majority of cancer patients being treated with conventional therapies (such as chemotherapy) experience awful side effects that dramatically decrease their quality of life. I believe we have the power to change that.

Every time my mom meets someone in the cancer hospital waiting room, she shares the story of how well the cannabis and mushrooms have been working for my dad's quality of life during his pancreatic cancer treatment. She frequently tells me stories of the people she meets, and how their eyes light up when they hear of these "supplements" that seem to be helping my dad so much. I love that my mom has become a beacon of hope and positivity for them during a difficult time.

Since I began sharing about cannabis and medicinal mushrooms,

I've been receiving emails and messages on social media every week with personal stories. Often, I get questions from people who were just diagnosed—but as more time goes by, I'm hearing stories of success, from patients using cannabis and mushrooms in conjunction with conventional treatment. Tumor blood markers going down, chemo side effects being eliminated, and tumors shrinking in size. I even hear stories of clear scans, which is always the brightest and most heart-warming moment of my day.

My friend Ty was diagnosed with stage IV Hodgkin's lymphoma at twenty-three years old. On the day that he was officially declared cancer free, he told me his story.

"When I was first diagnosed," he said, "I thought, *I can't leave yet—I have things to do. People are depending on me. I can't just drop out of this race. I haven't even scratched the surface of this life!* I had to take a stand for myself and for the people I love. My family and friends were a big motivating factor for me to get better. I knew that if I was really determined to be here, I had to become an active participant in my healing."

Ty went to an oncologist, but was terrified to do chemotherapy.

"My fear of chemotherapy was so strong. They told me I'd lose my hair, I'd experience extreme nausea and fatigue, brain fog, impaired digestion, weight loss, neuropathy, and that the chemotherapy and radiation could lead to secondary cancers. That sort of primal fear and existential anxiety is unparalleled. There's nothing that comes close to it. I developed insomnia, staying up for days at a time just from sheer anxiety."

Because of his fear of chemotherapy and the side effects he might experience, he delayed getting conventional treatment for a year and tried dietary remedies—but his tumors continued to grow. "The cancer outpaced me," he said. Eventually he decided to try chemotherapy, but he also began researching the best ways he could support his body holistically during treatment.

"I thought, *No matter what, I'm just going to fortify my body throughout all of this,*" said Ty. "My research led me to mushrooms and cannabis. I already knew they had incredible medicinal properties, so they became the primary tools I used during treatment."

Ty began using about half a gram of Rick Simpson Oil every day, and taking additional 1:1 CBD-to-THC capsules. He was also eating cannabis edibles and taking a blend of medicinal mushrooms in tincture form. All of the mushrooms in this book were included in his blend—chaga, reishi, maitake, shiitake, lion's mane, cordyceps, and turkey tail.

"I would put mushroom powders and CBD oil into my smoothies and coffee every day during treatment—and I still do today."

When Ty started his chemotherapy treatments, he was on edge, waiting for the side effects—but they never came. His white blood cell count never dropped below average.

"I experienced zero side effects for the entire duration of my chemotherapy. The nurses were baffled. They were pulling on my hair. 'You have no pain? You're not vomiting? No nausea? You haven't lost any of your hair?'"

The nurses had never seen anybody tolerate it the way Ty did. He was gaining weight. He was getting stronger.

"Even though the cancer treatments are over now, I still take cannabis and medicinal mushrooms every day. This is my lifestyle now. I'm just so grateful to be able to experience life. The human body is amazing."

Today, Ty is studying to become a health coach, and he's committed to spreading a message of healing to as many people as possible. "So much of this life comes down to choice," he says. "The doors to healing are everywhere, if you're open to them."

Ty's story is one of many who are experiencing a reduction or elimination of chemotherapy side effects from using cannabis and mushrooms during cancer treatment.

The side effects of chemotherapy can often be debilitating for a cancer patient's quality of life. Some of the most common side effects include:

- Nausea
- Vomiting
- Pain
- Appetite loss
- Hair loss
- Weight loss
- Neuropathy (nerve pain/numbness)
- Fatigue
- Extreme sensitivity to cold temperatures
- A weakened immune system

For many chemotherapy patients, the side effects get worse with each treatment, and the patients have to take a break, switch treatments, or stop the chemotherapy altogether. Oftentimes, even if a chemotherapy drug is working to slow the growth or reduce tumors, the side effects are so debilitating that it makes it impossible for the patient to continue with the treatment.

Ever since Thanksgiving of 2017, I've been doing research to help my dad manage the side effects of chemotherapy treatments with diet, supplements, and other home remedies. If you've seen someone go through chemotherapy side effects, you know firsthand that every little tip counts.

At the time of this writing, my dad's pancreas tumor is stable and dormant, and the tumor on his liver has shrunk to half the size it was initially. He's experienced very few side effects from chemo and has been able to enjoy a fantastic quality of life—traveling, golfing, gardening, and smiling every day. His outlook is positive, and his energy is as high as it's ever been. He often feels tired for a couple of days after chemo, but for the most part, he feels great.

Today was a good day.

—*Ray Sansouci, every day during cancer treatment*

Before we get started with some of the tips on managing side effects, I want to mention what I believe to be one of the most important aspects of this journey—*my dad's attitude.* He has stayed consistently positive and optimistic throughout this whole process, and I believe this makes a huge difference. Keeping an outlook of hope and positivity, and surrounding yourself with other people who share that optimism, can be profoundly healing in itself.

At the cancer hospital, he's been receiving a chemotherapy treatment called Folfirinox every two weeks. He goes into the hospital on a Wednesday, gets the chemotherapy administered for a few hours, and goes home with a chemo pump attached through a port in his chest that was surgically inserted. He spends two days at home getting the chemotherapy drugs administered through his port, and then goes back into the hospital on Friday to have it removed. He then has about twelve days off until his next cycle. He has completed over fifty cycles at the time of this writing, over two years.

Numbers-wise, there's a pancreatic tumor blood marker called CA 19-9—that's the one I've been watching every time he gets bloodwork done. Every kind of cancer has its own tumor blood marker. Normal levels of CA 19-9 (in people without pancreatic cancer) are between 0 and 37. When my dad started treatments, his CA 19-9 level had sky-rocketed to 1810. His number has been on the decline with every appointment since, and at the time of this writing, it's at 17, the lowest it's been so far. The doctors say they don't use this number as a final word on what's happening with the cancer—they just use it as a reference, but we keep track of it.

All of the things I'll outline in the next section are being done *in addition* to the treatments and medications from my dad's cancer hospital—*not instead of.* Please run everything by your oncologist before starting any new protocols.

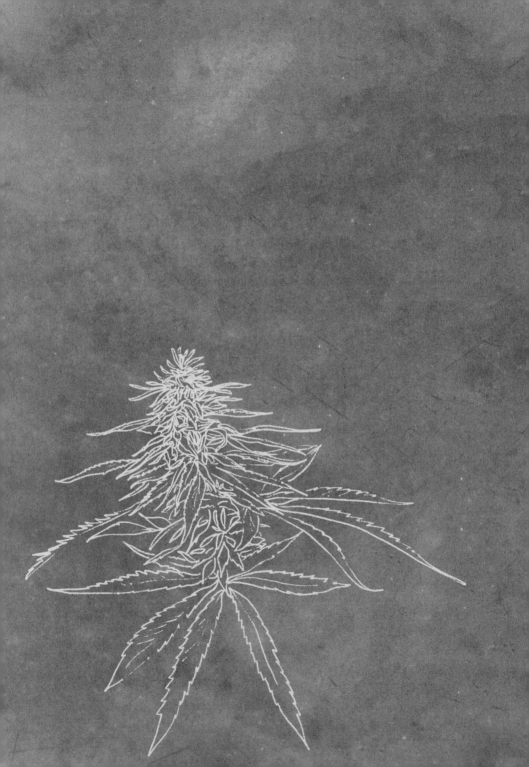

AT-HOME TIPS FOR MANAGING
CHEMO SIDE EFFECTS

This is the exact protocol my dad has been on. It is not a recommendation; it is simply for education and information. Remember, I'm not a doctor. . . . I'm just a girl who cares fiercely about her dad! It's not necessary to take all of these recommendations in order to alleviate your chemotherapy side effects—start with what you're inspired to start with and create a plan that works for you, your family, and your doctor. This is what we've been doing since the beginning, and since it seems to be working well, we haven't changed it.

FULL EXTRACT CANNABIS OIL (FECO)
OR RICK SIMPSON OIL (RSO)

This oil can help tremendously with nausea, sleep, appetite, pain, and mood. This high-potency cannabis oil comes in a needleless syringe, to be administered orally, and can be found at medical dispensaries. These oils are typically available in high-THC, high-CBD, and 1:1 ratios. The dose starts at the size of half a grain of rice, 2–3 times per day.

Increase dose slowly, as tolerated. Some cancer patients slowly work their way up to as much as 1 g per day. In a 1:1 ratio oil, this would equal 500 mg of CBD and 500 mg THC per day. My dad's dose is currently about one-fifth of that, or 100 mg CBD and 100 mg THC per day. Talk to a cannabis doctor or a medical dispensary budtender to help you find the right product for you.

CBD OIL

CBD oil is a great choice if you don't have access to medical cannabis. It can help ease pain and anxiety and help with sleep. In addition to the high-potency cannabis oil mentioned above, my dad takes 120 mg of full-spectrum CBD oil, in capsules, each day (two 30-mg capsules in the morning and two 30-mg capsules at night). He started taking these capsules before he got approved for his medical marijuana card, as they are federally legal to purchase online and at stores, and we wanted to get cannabinoids into his system as quickly as possible. He noticed such a significant reduction in joint pain from taking these capsules (he takes a brand called Wildflower) that he has continued with them even after getting his medical card and getting access to medical cannabis oil. This brings his total CBD intake to about 220 mg per day at the time of this writing, which is considered on the lower end for cancer dosing.

Medicinal Mushrooms

- **AHCC supplements.** My dad takes four 750-mg capsules of AHCC every day, for a total of 3 g per day (2 capsules in the morning and 2 at night). AHCC is a supplement derived from shiitake mushrooms. Studies have been done on AHCC for keeping the immune system strong during chemotherapy at amounts of 3 g per day.

- **Turkey tail mushrooms.** Currently, he is taking 2 g of turkey tail per day, in powder extract form (either in capsules or as powder mixed in a smoothie). When he's at home, he drinks a smoothie every day with a turkey tail powder extract added to it, and when traveling, he brings turkey tail capsules. Studies on turkey tail and cancer have shown it to be effective at enhancing immune cell function at doses of between 3 g and 9 g per day, so my dad's current dose is a conservative one.

- **A mushroom extract blend (powder) that includes chaga, reishi, lion's mane, maitake, shiitake, and cordyceps.** These extracts are available in powder, tincture, and capsule form. The typical dose in mushroom blends is about 150 mg of each mushroom, but studies have been done on medicinal mushrooms using much larger amounts, typically 1–5 g per day or more for a single mushroom—so again, my dad is taking a very conservative dose, and if we shift his protocol, I'll likely add larger amounts of all the other mushrooms. When you embark on an experiment with medicinal mushrooms, start with the recommended dose on the product you purchase and work your way up from there if desired.

- **Lion's mane mushrooms.** In addition to the mushroom blend, my dad takes 4 extra capsules of lion's mane daily, totaling 2 g per day, which has alleviated his chemotherapy-induced neuropathy.

MANAGING COMMON CHEMOTHERAPY SIDE EFFECTS

Nausea and Appetite Loss

Nausea and loss of appetite are two of the most common side effects of chemotherapy, and they can be a significant contributing factor to losing too much weight during cancer treatment.

Both CBD and THC have been shown to help with reducing nausea, and THC has been shown to stimulate appetite. A 1:1 CBD-to-THC cannabis oil can be tremendously helpful and is the main remedy my dad relies on. Because he has been on a steady stream of this cannabis oil every day, he hasn't had the need to use anything else for nausea or appetite. However, many chemotherapy patients report great success with inhalation (smoking or vaporizing with a dry herb vaporizer) or a CBD/THC oil tincture for nausea and appetite, too. Because inhalation and tinctures work so quickly, a dry herb vaporizer and CBD/THC oil tincture can be great options to have on hand for quick relief from acute bouts of nausea or appetite loss.

Change in Taste Buds

Another common side effect of chemotherapy is a change in taste buds—foods lack taste or change in taste completely, which means many chemo patients can no longer enjoy their favorite foods. As they likely already feel nauseated and without an appetite—and then food stops tasting good—this combination contributes to rapid weight loss in many patients. Chemotherapy drugs can really make it challenging to be able to eat, so we have to get creative.

There are a few things that can help, aside from the previously mentioned cannabis for appetite stimulation. One is a berry called the "miracle berry"—these berries make sour foods taste sweet, but they also change your taste buds (temporarily) in a way that can help make food taste good again. Many patients have reported being able to enjoy food after taking a miracle-berry tablet. You simply let the tablet dissolve on your tongue right before you eat your meal. Miracle-berry tablets are available to order online and are popular for "flavor tripping" (taking a miracle-berry tablet and then eating various foods to see how the flavors change—try it with a lemon or lime!) even in people who aren't undergoing chemotherapy.

> **Taste bud tip**: Many chemo patients report an unpleasant taste in their mouth when their port is flushed. (If you have a port, you'll know what I mean by this.) I recommend bringing honey/lemon lozenges to the hospital for the patient to suck on during port flushing, to make this more tolerable.

Jaw Pain

Jaw pain is another commonly reported chemotherapy side effect, which can make eating and chewing uncomfortable. Smoothies can be a game-changer when you lose your appetite, your taste buds change, or you're experiencing jaw pain that makes it hard to chew crunchy foods.

SUPERHERO SMOOTHIE

For patients who experience appetite loss, jaw pain, or loss of taste buds, it can often still be tolerable to drink a nutrient-rich shake. This is the smoothie that my mom makes for my dad every day. This smoothie helps my dad to get so many nutrients and calories into his system—greens, protein, antioxidants, healthy fats, and, of course, mushrooms! Sometimes I'll make a big batch of these smoothies and put them in freezer-safe jars, and put a few in the fridge (enough for two to three days) and a few in the freezer to save and thaw out when ready.

Don't worry about the exact amounts of each ingredient—play with what works for you. For patients who are sensitive to cold temperatures during chemotherapy, room-temperature smoothies are best.

Handful of spinach (or other greens, or a small scoop of greens powder)

1 banana or ½ avocado for creaminess

½ cup blueberries

1 cup almond milk, coconut milk, or water

1 Tbsp. almond butter or peanut butter

1 Tbsp. coconut oil

1–2 scoops protein powder (I like organic whey, pea, hemp, or collagen protein)

1 tsp. or more 10-mushroom blend powder (we use Four Sigmatic brand here)

1 tsp. or more turkey tail mushroom powder

Add everything to a blender, blend, and drink. Add more liquid (almond milk, coconut milk, or water) if necessary.

Bonus option: Add a dropperful of CBD oil to infuse some extra cannabinoids into your system.

A QUICK NOTE ON DIET AND CANCER

Everyone will have their opinion on the best cancer-fighting diet, and, of course, if your loved one on chemo is open to trying a specific diet (such as plant-based, vegan, paleo, or keto), do your research and go for it. I learned quickly that with my dad, since appetite and taste buds were scarce at the beginning and he was losing so much weight, I needed to focus on *adding* things in that he would enjoy and be able to stomach, to ensure he got enough healthy immune-boosting nutrients— rather than focusing on removing foods. Because of the nuances of appetite and taste buds during those first few months of chemo, we did not choose to embark on a specific elimination diet, aside from staying away from alcohol (completely) and sugar (reduced as much as possible). That's the way we've been doing things, and so far it works for him. This is such a personal journey, and everyone's food choices and food tolerability will be different. That being said, both holistic nutritionists and cancer hospital nutritionists will typically agree that reducing or eliminating sugar and alcohol are two of the most important things you can do, diet-wise, when battling cancer.

KRIS CARR'S GINGER AID JUICE

CONTRIBUTED BY KRIS CARR,
ORIGINALLY PUBLISHED IN *CRAZY SEXY JUICE*

My friend Kris was diagnosed with a rare, slow-growing form of stage IV cancer in 2003. She's been thriving with this cancer ever since, and she's dedicated her life to spreading a message of health and healing. She created a documentary based on her experience called *Crazy Sexy Cancer*, has written five best-selling books, and shares an abundance of tips on her website—not only for cancer, but for those interested in prevention and everyday wellness. Kris is the queen of green juices, and she's shared one of her nutrient-packed recipes with us here. As a bonus, the ginger happens to be great for nausea.

Makes 2 servings

½ cup spinach

1 large cucumber

2 celery stalks

1 large pear, cored

1-inch piece of ginger, peeled

Wash and prep all ingredients.

Juice all ingredients in a juicer, pour into two glasses, and serve.

Jenny's optional suggestions to make it "Rebel Style": add your preferred dose of CBD oil and/or a dropperful of chaga tincture, which can help soothe digestion. Stir into the juice.

CHEMO SIDE EFFECTS FOOD TIPS

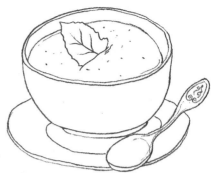

Make soups, stews, chilis, and broths. Any dish where you can add extra veggies, healthy fats, and protein that can be digested easily without having to chew through a big meal can help your loved one going through chemo get as many nutrients as possible. I've been making soups and chilis that are loaded with veggies, always adding extra chopped shiitake mushrooms, spinach, kale, celery, broccoli, or other vegetables to any recipe.

Bonus: When cooking for my dad, I *always* add a scoop of powdered turkey tail mushrooms to any savory dish.

Add-ins to soups, chilis, and broths for more nutrients, protein, and fat:

- Unflavored collagen powder

- Coconut oil (antiviral, great for the immune system)

- Avocado or avocado oil

- Greens—add extra spinach or kale into any savory dish

- Olive oil (drizzle your soup, stew, or chili with olive oil after it's done cooking—use your cannabis-infused oil here!)

- Unflavored CBD oil for extra cannabinoids—add into any meal

- Mushroom powder extracts of chaga, reishi, lion's mane, cordyceps, maitake, shiitake, or turkey tail—add to any meal

SLOW COOKER (OR INSTANT POT) TURKEY TAIL CHILI

I've been making different versions of this chili recipe a lot—changing it up as I like, adding different veggies.

You can make any chili recipe vegetarian or vegan by using more lentils (or other beans) instead of turkey or beef.

Makes 6 servings

To make this recipe paleo, eliminate the lentils. Either way, I always add a scoop of turkey tail powder! You can also make this in an Instant Pot rather than a slow cooker, I've provided those directions at the end of the recipe.

1 lb. ground turkey or grass-fed beef (leave this out to make it vegetarian)

1 Tbsp. olive oil

1 yellow onion, diced

2 cloves garlic, minced

Sea salt to taste

2 Tbsp. tomato paste

1 cup dry lentils (leave this out to make it paleo)

2 cups water

1 8-oz. can tomato sauce

1 14.5-oz. can diced tomatoes

1 4-oz. can diced green chilies

1 cup chopped mushrooms (shiitake or maitake)

2 cups chopped fresh spinach or kale

2 tsp. chili powder

1 tsp. cumin

1 Tbsp. or more turkey tail mushroom powder

1 tsp. pepper

Cilantro, chopped green onions, and slices of lime, for garnish (optional)

SLOW COOKER VERSION:

Add ground turkey or grass-fed beef and olive oil to a skillet over medium heat.

Add in the onion, garlic, and salt to taste. Cook until the meat is browned and onion is soft.

Add the mixture to your slow cooker.

Add lentils, water, tomato sauce, diced tomatoes, green chilies, mushrooms, spinach or kale, chili powder, cumin, turkey tail, and pepper to the slow cooker.

Cover and cook on high for 2–3 hours or on low for 4–6 hours, or until lentils are soft.

Scoop into serving bowls and top with cilantro, chopped green onions, and a squeeze of lime, if desired.

INSTANT POT VERSION:

Turn your pot to "sauté" and brown the turkey or beef.

Add in onion, garlic, and salt and cook until onion is soft.

Add the rest of the ingredients (except the garnishes).

Set your Instant Pot to "manual," cover, and set timer to 15 minutes.

When timer goes off, open the pressure valve to "venting" to release steam.

Once this is done, remove the lid and add chili to bowls. Top with optional cilantro, green onions, and lime juice.

HERO'S JOURNEY BONE BROTH

Another healing dish I love making is bone broth, which you can make in a slow cooker. Bone broth has been known to help with digestion, gut healing, skin, the immune system, hormonal health, joint pain, and more. It can give you a pep in your step and a sparkle in your eye when you're feeling under the weather. This bone broth recipe uses two different kinds of wonderful, health-enhancing mushrooms. If you're looking for a vegetarian broth recipe, check out Marco Canora's Shiitake Mushroom Broth on page 158.

2–4 lbs. meat or poultry bones (ask your friendly local butcher!)

4 qts. water (or just enough water to cover everything)

1 tsp. sea salt

2 Tbsp. apple cider vinegar

1 large onion, coarsely chopped

5–7 cloves garlic, chopped or lightly smashed

1 cup chopped, fresh stemmed shiitake mushrooms (or ½ cup dried)

1 cup chopped, fresh maitake mushrooms (or ½ cup dried)

10 (or so) leaves of fresh sage

2–3 inches fresh ginger, peeled and chopped

A few shakes of freshly ground black pepper

If you're using beef bones, you'll want to roast them before you put them in the pot to make broth. This gives the broth a much better flavor. Put bones into a roasting dish and roast at 400°F for 30 minutes, or until nicely browned.

Place all ingredients in a large slow cooker and set on high.

Bring to a simmer (this may take a few hours), then reduce the setting to low for 12–24 hours (or more). I usually take mine off at about 24 hours, but you can go longer if you want it to taste richer. Strain the broth through a strainer into a large bowl or large mason jars and compost the bones/vegetables (unless you want to use the bones again for another pot of broth, which you can). If you don't have a slow cooker you can still make this recipe on a stovetop, with a large pot on low heat.

When you've strained out the broth, put it in the fridge until the fat rises to the top. Then scrape the fat off with a spoon and discard it before reheating the broth to drink it. (Some people keep the fat to cook veggies with; you can do that if you want to, as long as you aren't using bones from conventionally raised animals. There are likely to be more toxins stored in the fat of conventionally raised animals.)

Drink bone broth from a mug—as many mugs as you like. You can add it to soups and other recipes for nutrition and flavor. You can keep the bone broth in the fridge for 3–4 days or in the freezer for up to a year. But I guarantee it won't last that long! You can also freeze your bone broth in ice cube trays and easily pop a broth cube into any soup, stew, stir-fry, or other dish you're cooking.

COLD SENSITIVITY AND NEUROPATHY

Cold sensitivity and tingling fingers and toes (due to neuropathy) are common experiences when undergoing chemotherapy. Neuropathy is common with most chemotherapy drugs, but the cold sensitivity is usually associated with a chemotherapy drug called Oxaliplatin. If you have this cold sensitivity, make sure you have a good set of gloves on hand, especially if you're going through chemo in the winter. Reaching into the refrigerator may require gloves, too—so keep a pair near the fridge. It's important to keep a jug of room-temperature drinking water nearby at all times so you can stay hydrated without feeling pain from cold water.

For cold winter months, or times when you're extra-sensitive to cold during chemo, consider getting an infrared heating mat. My dad has been sitting on his mat every day, and it's been warming him up through the cold winter months. Infrared heating mats are also reported to have immune-boosting effects.

Neuropathy typically shows up as tingling, "pins and needles," pain, or numbness in the hands and feet. Lion's mane mushroom can be helpful for this type of neuropathy as it can regenerate myelin, which protects nerve fibers. Neuropathy in the fingertips, along with being painful, can make it hard for chemotherapy patients to do things like button buttons and feel things properly with their fingers, which lion's mane may help to improve. A typical dose of lion's mane is 1–3 g daily.

GENERAL IMMUNE SYSTEM HEALTH

Along with the specific symptoms that come along with chemotherapy, it's extremely important to keep the immune system strong. Chemotherapy drugs can weaken the immune system, which can make you more likely to catch a cold or get sick during your treatment. The best remedy here is to support the immune system as much as possible, so you can stay feeling healthy while the chemo does its job of fighting the cancer. All of the medicinal mushrooms in this book are specifically geared toward this purpose, to keep the immune system healthy. As we have cannabinoid receptors in our immune system, using cannabis therapeutically also has great potential for immune system support. In addition to medicinal mushrooms and cannabis, turn back to the Upgrade Your Immunity chapter for a list of some of my favorite immune system supporters.

TIPS FOR CAREGIVERS

If you're caring for someone you love while they go through cancer treatments, taking care of yourself is one of the greatest gifts you can give them. One of my blog readers emailed me this tip when I first started sharing about our journey:

"REMEMBER—YOUR OWN WELL-BEING IS SO IMPORTANT TO THE OVERALL GOAL."

When you're taking care of someone else, your own health and well-being can be all too easy to let slide as your priorities shift. But the more time you take to nurture your own health, the more you'll be able to be there for the person you love who is going through treatment. Stay rested and hydrated, get enough exercise, eat nourishing foods, and keep some form of social and spiritual connection strong. Your immune system, energy, and attitude will make a huge difference in your loved one's experience and healing process. Don't ever feel guilty about taking immaculate care of yourself.

When someone is sick, that person tends to get most of the focus and attention. With all of the appointments, medications, trips to the hospital, and day-to-day care, it can be tough to focus on your own well-being. My mom has been a powerful example for me. She has made a point to stay optimistic, strong, and full of light, never skimping on her own self-care (taking long walks, eating healthy meals, drinking lots of green tea, and prioritizing sleep) through this process. This has absolutely contributed to my dad's well-being, and the well-being of my sister and me, too.

If you're helping someone who's going through treatment to get on an immune-boosting supplement regimen, or making them a smoothie or nourishing meal, make sure to save some for yourself, too.

I know how incredibly challenging it can be to stay strong and vibrant during these times, but do your best to keep your hope alive and your spirits up. There are miracle stories and positive outcomes that happen every day. Focus on those. Share stories of hope and healing with your loved one. Stay present for every conversation and moment you share together along the way. Although this is likely one of the greatest challenges you will ever face in your life, there are ways to make it more manageable, and find some beauty, wisdom, and joy in these precious life moments together.

Life becomes a little more vivid and brilliant when you go through things like this. You appreciate everything so much more.

—Nancy Sansouci (my mom)

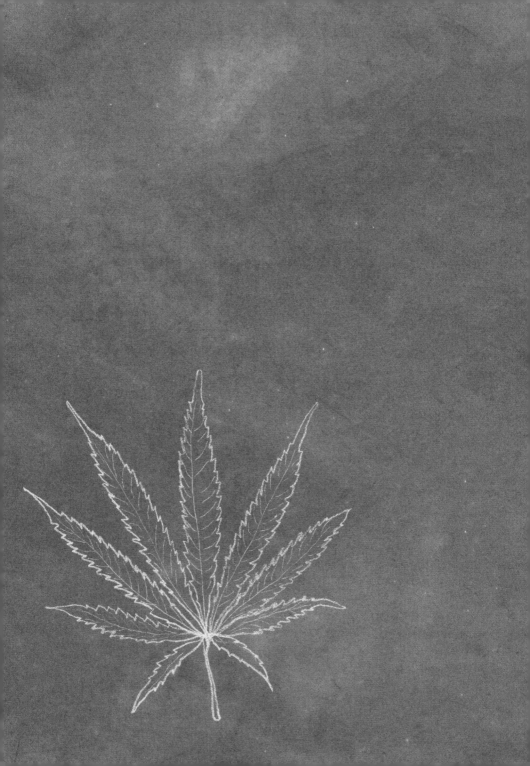

OTHER ADVANCED CASES

Because cannabis and medicinal mushrooms can have an incredible array of applications for health, there are many different conditions that tend to respond well to them. We have cannabinoid receptors that interact with cannabis molecules throughout every system in the body, and as you've seen already, medicinal mushrooms are powerhouses for the immune system. Both cannabis and mushrooms help to keep our bodies in homeostasis (balance), so depending on your condition, they could be a worthy addition to your treatment regimen with your doctor's consent. Again, remember that every person is different, so monitor your progress closely and keep a journal to record your dosage and any effects that you feel.

When working with cannabis and advanced conditions, dosing can take some experimentation, and I always recommend working directly with a cannabis doctor. To find a cannabis doctor near you, do an online search for "medical cannabis doctor" and your specific city—or visit the Society of Cannabis Clinicians at cannabisclinicians.org. Some cannabis doctors offer online video consultations if you can't make it face-to-face.

When using medicinal mushrooms to help with an advanced condition, it would be wise to work with a naturopathic doctor or alternative health practitioner who has experience with using medicinal mushrooms. Typically, dosing with medicinal mushrooms for advanced conditions is about five times the recommended standard wellness dose.

Here are a few examples of conditions that are showing promise for treatment with cannabis or mushrooms:

Epilepsy. The popular CBD oil company Charlotte's Web was named after a little girl named Charlotte Figi, who developed Dravet syndrome—a form of epilepsy that produces constant seizures—when she was a baby. By the time she was three years old, she was having about 300 seizures a week—and according to her mom, Paige, she sometimes experienced more than 50 seizures in one night. The first day Charlotte took CBD oil under her tongue, she had no seizures that day. She had no seizures for the following few days, either, when, according to her mom in the CNN documentary *Weed*, "she would have normally had one hundred." According to a 2019 article in *The New York Times*, Charlotte continues to be almost entirely seizure-free.

Since then, many other patients have used CBD successfully for seizures, and a CBD-isolate pharmaceutical drug called Epidiolex (prescribed for seizure disorders) was approved by the FDA in 2018. Researchers have found, however, that full-spectrum CBD is three times as effective as the single-molecule drug for seizure disorders. Full-spectrum CBD oil also produced fewer unwanted side effects than the isolate.

PTSD. Studies have shown that patients experiencing post-traumatic stress disorder (PTSD) symptoms have low levels of anandamide (one of the endogenous cannabinoids), and that there are cannabinoid receptors located on the amygdala in the brain—which is associated with anxiety, fear response, and memory retrieval. Many PTSD patients report a reduction in their symptoms when using cannabis therapeutically.

MAPS (Multidisciplinary Association for Psychedelic Studies) is currently training therapists to guide patients through MDMA (the active compound in the drug ecstasy) therapy for PTSD. In Phase 2 clinical trials, 68 percent of participants no longer met the criteria for a PTSD diagnosis one year following MDMA treatment. Phase 3 trials are currently under way. MDMA doesn't come from cannabis or mushrooms—but it's worth keeping your finger on the pulse of this research if you suffer from PTSD.

Alzheimer's, Parkinson's, multiple sclerosis, and other neurological conditions. Both cannabis and lion's mane mushroom have been shown to be neuroregenerative and potentially therapeutic for conditions related to the brain and nerves. Cannabinoids have been shown to be neuroprotective, potentially reducing the progression of neurological conditions. In MS specifically, a 1:1 ratio of CBD to THC has been shown to reduce pain and spasticity. Researchers are studying psilocybin mushrooms for their neuroregenerative properties as well.

Autoimmune conditions. Many autoimmune conditions involve an inflammatory response in the body; reducing inflammation can often help to tame symptoms. We have CB1 and CB2 cannabinoid receptors located on our immune cells, and cannabis has been shown to help modulate the immune system and calm inflammation. Medicinal mushrooms have all been shown to help modulate (rather than stimulate) the immune system and can potentially help with autoimmune conditions.

"If you have an autoimmune condition or if you are on medication for an autoimmune disease, I recommend working with a naturopath, a medical doctor or nurse practitioner who's knowledgeable about herbs, a very experienced herbalist, or other practitioners who are knowledgeable about autoimmune disease medications and botanicals," says Aviva Romm, MD.

Treatment-resistant depression. Psilocybin mushrooms are currently being studied with patients experiencing severe depression that has failed to respond to other treatments. Psilocybin has been given a "breakthrough therapy" designation by the FDA, to accelerate clinical trials and drug development. Breakthrough therapy status is typically granted when preliminary evidence indicates that a drug may demonstrate substantial improvement over other available therapies, according to the FDA. Clinical trials with psilocybin are currently under way. (More on psilocybin in the next section.)

Visit RebelsApothecary.com/Resources for the latest research and updates on cannabis, mushrooms, and health conditions. ProjectCBD.org also offers many of the latest updates on cannabis science and research for a wide variety of different conditions.

MAGIC MUSHROOMS:
THE CASE FOR PSILOCYBIN

My life's mission is to advance legal psychedelic therapy," said Rick Doblin, executive director of the Multidisciplinary Association for Psychedelic Studies (MAPS), at a talk my dad and I attended together at Harvard Business School. "We're all suffering with fears, anxieties, and low levels of trauma. There's a need for mass mental health."

Also presenting at the event was George Goldsmith, co-founder of COMPASS Pathways—a company that's currently positioned to become the first legal provider of psilocybin (the psychedelic compound in magic mushrooms) for treatment-resistant depression. In 2018 COMPASS Pathways was granted "breakthrough therapy" designation from the FDA to run the first large-scale clinical trials with psilocybin, which are currently under way.

All of the medicinal mushrooms we've covered so far in *The Rebel's Apothecary* have been non-psychedelic, although you probably noticed that I mentioned psilocybin mushrooms briefly a few times. The medicinal mushrooms we've covered up until now can do many powerful things, but "magic mushrooms" are truly in a class of their own. The budding research on psilocybin could completely revolutionize the way we approach mental health care.

Psilocybin is currently being studied for its potential as a frontline treatment for a variety of conditions, including depression, anxiety, PTSD, addiction, smoking cessation, obsessive-compulsive disorder (OCD), and alcohol dependence. A very telling sign of the times, two major psychedelic research centers just opened in 2019—the Johns Hopkins Center for Psychedelic and Consciousness Research, and the Centre for Psychedelic Research at Imperial College London. Entrepreneur and author Tim Ferriss, who has been vocal on his podcast about supporting psychedelic research, played a role in the funding for both centers. We're just at the beginning of a psychedelic renaissance, and the next few years should bring major changes in research, progress, and legalization.

WHAT IS A MAGIC MUSHROOM?

The definition of "magic mushroom" in the dictionary says, "any toadstool with hallucinogenic properties." The word "toadstool" makes me smile. A magic mushroom, to put it simply, is any mushroom that can produce psychedelic effects. Psilocybin is the psychedelic compound found in a category of fungi known as "psilocybe" mushrooms, and there are over 180 varieties. Psilocybin has traditionally been used in healing rituals and spiritual ceremonies throughout many different cultures, and ancient cave drawings of these magic mushrooms date back thousands of years.

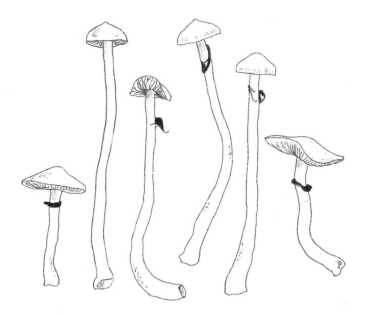

CURRENT PSILOCYBIN RESEARCH

Research on psilocybin was halted in the late 1960s as it became associated with the counterculture, and psilocybin was deemed a Schedule 1 illegal drug (the same classification as cannabis) under the Controlled Substances Act of 1970.

While psilocybin is still classified as Schedule 1 in the United States, the research happening today will likely shift legality in the coming years. In fact, some cities (including Denver and Oakland) are beginning to decriminalize psilocybin. "Decriminalization" means that although it's still illegal, it's considered the lowest law enforcement priority, and money won't be spent to carry out criminal penalties around it.

The research on psilocybin began to reemerge in the 1990s, as the FDA gave the green light to some research institutions to continue psychedelic research in humans. Researchers at Johns Hopkins have been studying psilocybin ever since, and many other studies are emerging. Research is accelerating now, and so far, results are exciting and promising.

COMPASS Pathways recently released their preliminary findings from phase 1 clinical trials at King's College London, finding psilocybin safe for consumption and showing no adverse events in their participants. Phase 2 trials will include data from a larger population of patients experiencing treatment-resistant depression.

The opening of new psychedelic research centers around the world will continue to advance the potential therapeutic uses for psilocybin. At Imperial College London, a study is currently running to compare the antidepressant effects of psilocybin to SSRIs (selective serotonin reuptake inhibitors), which are the most commonly prescribed type of pharmaceutical antidepressant. "Here at the center for psychedelic research, we're passionate about improving mental health care at a time when it is so desperately needed. We're hopeful about bringing a deeper, more human, holistic quality of care to those who suffer," says Robin Carhart-Harris, head of the Centre for Psychedelic Research at Imperial College London.

In a 2016 study on psilocybin in cancer patients led by Dr. Roland Griffiths at Johns Hopkins University, a single dose of psilocybin produced substantial and enduring decreases in depression and anxiety, along with increases in life meaning and optimism. At a six-month follow-up, these changes were sustained.

The psilocybin sessions, which usually last about six hours, take place in a comfortable, living room–like setting rather than a clinical doctor's office. The participant lies on a couch with an eye mask and headphones on, listening to soothing music under the supervision of a trained guide. Often, participants report having deeply mystical experiences.

"These experiences are characterized by a sense of unity, a feeling that all people and things are connected, accompanied by a sense of sacredness, a sense of positive mood, love, joy, and a deeply felt sense of encountering ultimate reality," said Dr. Roland Griffiths in a 2016 TEDMED talk. "Long-term follow-up shows that these positive effects are sustained for at least a year, and probably longer."

HOW DOES PSILOCYBIN WORK?

Psilocybin is metabolized in the body into a compound called psilocin, which binds to serotonin 5-HT2A receptors in the brain—these receptors play a role in mood regulation. Experts say psilocybin deactivates what they call the "default mode network"—the part of the brain associated with rumination and sense of self (often referred to as ego)—and can help the brain form new neurological pathways. Based on reports from study participants, psilocybin sessions can lead to substantial perspective shifts, disruption in patterns of negative thinking, and profound mystical experiences. More research on the exact mechanisms in the brain is still needed—this research will continue to develop in the coming years.

PSILOCYBIN DOSES IN RESEARCH

All of the studies on psilocybin are being done in guided therapeutic environments, and the doses being used are larger than a typical "recreational" magic mushroom dose. For reference, the amounts used in these studies are equal to roughly 3–5 g of dried psilocybin mushrooms, considered a highly psychedelic dose. A recreational or social dose (that someone might take at a party or festival, for example) is typically less—often between .5 and 2 g. With psilocybin, even a 1-g increase in dose can make a big difference in the intensity of the psychedelic effects. While a lighter dose may bring pleasant sensory enhancement and mind expansion (while still allowing you to interact with the outside world), just 1 extra gram could take you on a full psychedelic "trip." Psychedelic writer and pioneer Terence McKenna famously coined 5 g of psilocybin as a "heroic dose"—typically an intense experience producing strong hallucinations and a deep dive into the inner workings of the psyche. For these reasons, it's important not to experiment with psilocybin by yourself, and to do so only under the care of a trained psychedelic therapist.

MICRODOSING PSILOCYBIN

The studies mentioned on psilocybin are being conducted with large, psychedelic doses—but what about microdosing? Microdosing, or taking a tiny, "subperceptual" amount of a psychedelic compound, has seen a recent rise in popularity among both people suffering from depression or anxiety, and productivity-minded creatives and entrepreneurs. Microdosing has been reported to help with stress, anxiety, depression, and cluster headaches, and many people who microdose say they use it for focus, mental clarity, energy, and creativity.

According to Dana Larsen of the Medicinal Mushroom Dispensary, a typical dose of psilocybin mushrooms for psychedelic purposes is between 1 and 3 g of the dried mushroom. A microdose, he says, is much smaller—between 1 percent and 10 percent of an active dose. This means a microdose of psilocybin mushrooms can range anywhere from the tiniest bit (.01 g) to about .3 g of the dried mushroom.

Anything above .5 g is typically considered a psychedelic dose. If you are experimenting with microdosing (again, it is not recommended to experiment with any psychedelic without a trained therapist or guide), starting as low as possible is the safest bet (just like with cannabis dosing). The effects of a microdose last for 4–6 hours, so if you take too much, you'll have to wait it out, which may feel unpleasant if you were expecting the effects to be subperceptual.

Some consider a starter microdose to be around .10 g, though those who are completely new to psychedelics (or sensitive in general) often start with even lower amounts.

"We strongly suggest starting with the lowest possible dose and working your way upwards," say Virginia Haze and Dr. K. Mandrake, PhD, in *The Psilocybin Mushroom Bible*. "If it's too little and you don't feel anything, you've lost nothing; your day has just been as it would have been anyway."

What Does Microdosing Feel Like?

The term "subperceptual" means you shouldn't experience any psychedelic effects or notice much of a difference in perception at all. Although everyone is different, most people who microdose with psilocybin report an elevated mood, along with feeling focused, clear, and creative. You may feel more present and attuned to the moment. You may find that negative stories or emotions that usually bog you down will be lifted away. Answers to questions or problems might seem more obvious than they did before. You may find yourself having subtle revelations, realizations, or epiphanies, but you shouldn't experience any hallucinations. If you've taken the "right" microdose, you may just feel like you . . . but slightly enhanced.

How Often Do People Microdose?

Many microdosing enthusiasts report using either the Fadiman Protocol, the Stamets Protocol, or their own personal protocol.

James Fadiman, author of *The Psychedelic Explorer's Guide*, recommends a microdosing protocol of one microdose every three days—meaning one day on, then two days off, then one day on, and so forth.

On podcast episode #1385 of *The Joe Rogan Experience*, mushroom expert Paul Stamets, who recently launched a microdosing app, recommended a protocol of four days on, three days off.

These protocols are just suggestions, however. Some people prefer to microdose more or less often, depending on their response to it. You can still feel the "afterglow" of a microdose the next day—typically a gentle, pleasant feeling.

"Microdosing below the threshold of intoxication benefits neurogenesis," says Stamets. "It has enormous potential." Neurogenesis refers to the formation of new neurons in the brain.

How Is a Microdose Measured?

Those who happen to acquire magic mushrooms often use a small digital scale to weigh out a microdose with their dried mushrooms. Some people like to grind their mushrooms (in a coffee grinder, or with a mortar and pestle) and measure specific amounts of powder into capsules. This helps to make sure the active compound psilocybin is evenly distributed, as some parts of the mushroom may contain more psilocybin than others. Some people simply bite off a piece of a dried mushroom, but this makes the psilocybin distribution more uneven and difficult to measure.

Others choose to grind their psilocybin mushroom into a powder, measure out the microdose on a digital scale, and dissolve it into hot water to make tea.

Paul Stamets has spoken about the synergy between lion's mane and psilocybin for increased neurogenesis.

Other mycologists agree. "Taking lion's mane and psilocybin together is like piecing your brain back together," said Tradd Cotter at his medicinal mushroom seminar.

Hypothetically, if psilocybin becomes legal, you could consider making tea with lion's mane powder and adding a tiny microdose of psilocybin powder to it for an extra boost of brain power.

Who Shouldn't Consider Microdosing?

Psilocybin is illegal, so all of the information contained here is for informational purposes only. If you're in sober recovery, you'll likely want to steer clear of psilocybin, as it's a psychedelic compound. It's important to know that psilocybin could alter your perception a little bit even at small doses, and you could have a full-on psychedelic trip at larger doses.

According to James Fadiman's site, MicrodosingPsychedelics.com: "We specifically do not recommend that people who live with diagnoses of psychotic disorders or are along the autism spectrum try microdosing. People with colorblindness report lasting visual distortions from microdosing." If you have any concerns about the state of your mental or physical health and are considering microdosing, consult with a doctor or psychedelic therapist, and check out the Zendo Project for information on psychedelic harm reduction.

My Microdosing Experience

As I was in the process of researching for this book, I was listening to Michael Pollan's book *How to Change Your Mind* on audio. On a Saturday afternoon, as I was walking down the street listening to the book, my ears perked up as I heard him talking about the research going on with psilocybin mushrooms for depression.

Depression is something I've struggled with on and off throughout my life. If you've experienced depression yourself, you know it isn't always situational—it can come on regardless of life circumstance. To me, depression can feel physically crushing—I liken it to an elephant stepping on my chest. Even if I can rationally look around at my life and see that nothing's "wrong," when I'm feeling depressed, the elephant is there, squashing me into a pancake. This kind of depression can be incredibly hard to feel relief from.

On that particular afternoon, the elephant was there, smashing its heavy foot into my chest. I knew I could do some things that would help to alleviate it—I could breathe, I could meditate, I could exercise, I could call my sister or best friend, and some of it would lift, for sure. But in certain instances, regardless of what technique I try, the pressure is still there. As I listened to Michael Pollan describe how effective psilocybin has been shown to be for depression, something clicked. A few weeks prior, a friend of mine had gifted me "three microdoses" of psilocybin mushrooms. I had curiously accepted the gift and tucked it away in a secret place, and hadn't thought about it since. That day, however, I remembered the gift and decided to try just the tiniest amount. I took out my journal so I could record any differences in how I felt.

About fifteen minutes into my first microdose, I was astonished to feel that *the elephant was stepping off of my chest*. The smushed, suffocated depression feeling started to lift. I could actually physically feel the relief, as the emotional burden I was carrying, which sometimes feels all-consuming, began to evaporate. I understood immediately why they were using psilocybin in studies for depression. I didn't feel any psychedelic "tripping" effects—I just felt the elephant go away. I was able to do all the normal things I was planning to do that evening— clean up my apartment, cook dinner, write . . . but the elephant had left the building. I felt lighter, clearer, and much less bogged down by the weight of my thoughts.

That first experience was enough for me to be a believer in microdosing for depression. Once my mood had lifted, I was able to notice other interesting effects from microdosing—primarily, an increase in focus and concentration. As I was cooking dinner, I found myself *noticing every little detail* of my food. I cut into a blood orange and gasped out loud at how beautiful it looked. It was a deep ruby red and orange color, it almost looked tie-dyed, and it was shimmering slightly in the light of my kitchen. I admired it for much longer than I normally would when cutting into an orange. Since then, I've come to learn that color and light are two of the most noticeable perceptual changes that occur when you take a small amount of psilocybin. Even without experiencing hallucinations or a psychedelic trip, lights look brighter, and details look finer. Some people report that they experience "HD vision" when they microdose. Under the influence of the tiny bit of psilocybin, I felt like I could see things clearly for what they really were, instead of through the lens of my own old and familiar stories. It was a subtle but obvious sensation. I could simply be present and appreciate the beauty around me, with much more vibrant detail.

Microdoses of psilocybin have continued to support me, on and off, ever since. As you know, I have no interest in feeling high or disoriented, and I generally need way less than a typical microdose to feel my mood lift and the focusing effects kick in. I can feel mood elevation from just the tiniest bit of a psilocybin mushroom. We're talking about a piece of a mushroom the size of a small chili flake—usually between .01 and .05 g, but sometimes so small it doesn't even register on the scale. Obviously, this is considered a very tiny microdose, but I still receive the benefits.

Personally, I don't think microdosing psilocybin is *completely* sub-perceptual. I always notice tiny shifts in perception, even if it's just colors looking a little more vibrant or lights looking a little brighter. But compared to what it felt like to do large doses of magic mushrooms (in which case the entire world looks completely different, or even disappears), a microdose barely registers, and life goes on as normal—just subtly enhanced.

THE IMPORTANCE OF SET, SETTING, AND INTENTION

You may have heard of the concept "set and setting" as it relates to psychedelics. "Set" refers to your mindset when you embark on an experiment with psychedelics, and "setting" is the environment you're in, and who is around you. All of this is very important if you want to have a healthy, therapeutic experience. There's a reason the psilocybin experiments are being done in a relaxed living-room setting—so participants can feel as comfortable as possible. Your intention is important as well. If you find yourself curious about psychedelic therapy, take some time to write down why you're drawn to psychedelics and what you hope to get from the experience. As psychedelic therapy expands in the coming years, you may soon have access to psilocybin in a guided, therapeutic setting.

I'm excited to see where the future of psilocybin research and treat-

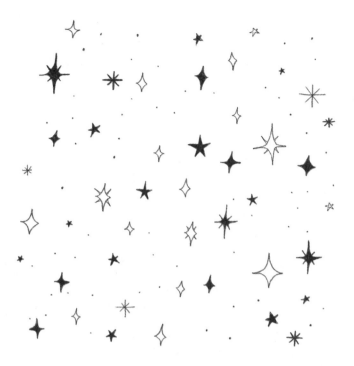

ment is heading. Most experts in the field predict that in the coming years, psilocybin will become legal for use in a therapy setting, but not legal to simply purchase at a store. This seems logical, so patients can be monitored and appropriate safety measures can be taken.

We'll be seeing more from psilocybin, and psychedelics in general, as studies continue to unfold, and legalization continues to shift. This is just the beginning.

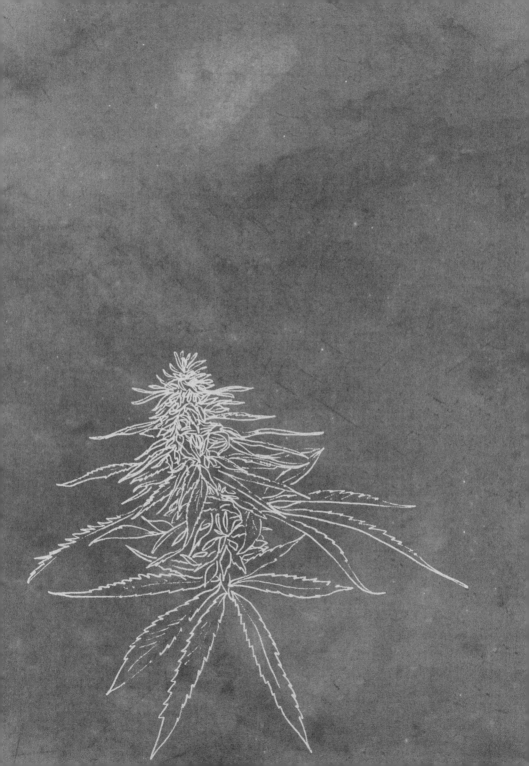

CREATING YOUR OWN REBEL'S APOTHECARY

**Plants have amazing powers . . . they are
filled with so much wonder.**

—Paul Tappenden

Now that you've reached the end of the book, you're completely stocked with information and research to help you get started on your own healing journey with cannabis and mushrooms—along with other plants, herbs, recipes, and supportive lifestyle practices. Build your apothecary slowly. Try one remedy at a time. Keep a journal to record anything new that you try. Enjoy the experience of going to a dispensary for the first time and reveling in the fact that you can now have an informed conversation with the lovely budtenders. Go to your local herb shop. Look around, ask questions. See if they have any medicinal mushrooms there, like dried reishi, or wild-harvested chaga. Make teas. Try a tincture. Start to deepen your relationship with natural remedies from the Earth. Stay curious as you get to know exactly what works for you, your body, and your life. Your world is about to become richer and more expansive, as you courageously travel down the rebel's path.

Having confidence in the healing power of nature, and spreading that message, is the most important thing you can do.

—Dr. Andrew Weil, speaking at the
2019 Integrative Nutrition Conference

The resources listed on the next page will help you get started with creating your own home apothecary. Thank you for taking this journey with me!

RESOURCES

UPDATED RESOURCES CAN BE FOUND AT
REBELSAPOTHECARY.COM/RESOURCES.

CANNABIS LAWS AND REFORM

NORML (National Organization for the Reform of Marijuana Laws):
norml.org

Americans for Safe Access: safeaccessnow.org

Drug Policy Alliance: drugpolicy.org

CANNABIS EDUCATION

Healer.com

ProjectCBD.org

Leafly.com

WeedMaps.com

MUSHROOM PRODUCTS AND EDUCATION

Mushroom Clubs: North American Mycological Association

Catskill Fungi

Mushroom Mountain/MycoMatrix

Four Sigmatic

SuperFeast

Fungi Perfecti/Host Defense

Nammex

Real Mushrooms

North Spore

A FEW LAB-TESTED CBD OILS I USE AND LOVE

SupHERBals

Care By Design

Papa & Barkley

Lazarus Naturals

Wildflower Brands

Charlotte's Web

OTHER CANNABIS BRANDS I LOVE

Foria (broad-spectrum CBD and suppositories)

Mary's Medicinals (1:1 transdermal compound)

Apothecanna (body oil)

Fields of Hemp (CBD flower)

HERB AND SUPPLEMENT DRUG INTERACTIONS

Memorial Sloan Kettering Cancer Center (mskcc.org: search for the supplement or herb you're curious about in the search box at the top of the site)

HERBAL MEDICINE INFORMATION

Mountain Rose Herbs

American Botanical Council: abc.herbalgram.org

Medicinal Herbs: A Beginner's Guide by Rosemary Gladstar

CANNABIS BOOKS

Smoke Signals by Martin A. Lee

The Cannabis Manifesto by Steve DeAngelo

CBD: A Patient's Guide to Medicinal Cannabis by Leonard Leinow and Julia Birnbaum

Cannabis Revealed by Bonni Goldstein, M.D.

Cannabis Pharmacy by Michael Backes

The Leafly Guide to Cannabis by the Leafly Team

Rick Simpson Oil: Nature's Cure for Cancer by Rick Simpson

MUSHROOM BOOKS

The Fungal Pharmacy by Robert Rogers

Organic Mushroom Farming and Mycoremediation by Tradd Cotter

Mycelium Running by Paul Stamets

Mycophilia by Eugenia Bone

Chaga: King of the Medicinal Mushrooms by David Wolfe

Medicinal Mushrooms by Christopher Hobbs

Healing Mushrooms by Tero Isokauppila

Growing Gourmet and Medicinal Mushrooms by Paul Stamets

Fantastic Fungi by Paul Stamets

A Field Guide to Medicinal Mushrooms of North America by Daniel Winkler and Robert Rogers

OTHER BOOKS AND EDUCATIONAL RESOURCES

How to Change Your Mind by Michael Pollan

The Psilocybin Mushroom Bible by Virginia Haze and Dr. K. Mandrake, PhD

The International Journal of Medicinal Mushrooms

Fungi Magazine

FILMS

Fantastic Fungi

Weed the People

Run from the Cure

PSYCHEDELIC EDUCATION

MAPS.org

Heffter.org

MichaelPollan.com/Resources

ACKNOWLEDGMENTS

To anyone who has ever written a book: I am in awe of you. I had no idea what it would take to complete a project of this scope—but if you're reading this it means I finished it, which is unbelievable news.

So many people contributed to this book coming to life:

To my wonderful agent, Stephanie Tade, thank you for not only being a teammate but a dear friend. Thank you to Colleen Martell, for your feedback on my ideas and proposal. Michelle Garside, for igniting the initial spark that became this book. Thank you to my exceptional editor, Marian Lizzi, and the whole TarcherPerigee team at Penguin Random House: Rachel Ayotte, Allyssa Fortunato, Sara Johnson, Roshe Anderson, Anne Kosmoski, Megan Newman, Lindsay Gordon, Lorie Pagnozzi, Joel Breuklander, and Anne Chan. Thank you to Basak Notz for your gorgeous botanical illustrations.

Janna Hockenjos—thank you (and Cam) for your genius edits, and for talking me off the ledge with deep yoga breaths when it got hard. Richelle Fredson—thank you for your supportive guidance every step of the way, from book proposal to published book. Miles Rote—the light, enthusiasm, and unconditional support you poured into this entire project, and my process, was otherworldly. I am deeply grateful.

Special thanks to Martin A. Lee, Dr. Ethan Russo, John Michelotti, Dr. Dustin Sulak, and Professor Solomon P. Wasser for your generous fact-checking, contributions, and support.

Thank you to all of the amazing recipe contributors—Kris Carr, Chris Herko, Amanda Carney, Olga Cotter, Marco Canora, Seamus Mullen, Robyn Youkilis, Matcha Kari, Dr. Jeremy Goldberg, Kendra Adachi, Will Hickox, and Janna and Chad Hockenjos. Thank you to Ty Decaires, for sharing your story.

To Greg Prasker, Cheryl Boiko, Jo Anne Richards, Tradd Cotter, Paul Stamets, Raphael Mechoulam, Dr. Andrew Weil, Tero Isokauppila, David Wolfe, Dr. Annemarie Colbin, Rick Simpson, Eugenia Bone, Leonard Leinow, Dr. Bonni Goldstein, Steve D'Angelo, Dr. Aviva Romm, Rosemary Gladstar, Robert Rogers, Daniel Winkler, Tim Ferriss, Rick Doblin, Dr. Robin Carhart-Harris, Dr. Roland Griffths, and Michael Pollan, thank you for your work that has taught me so much. I look forward to spending the rest of my life in relationship with medicinal plants. Thank you to Project CBD, Canna-Craft, the CannMed Conference, Catskill Fungi, Mushroom Mountain, and Remedies Herb Shop for being instrumental parts of my learning process.

Thank you to Brooklyn Yoga Project (and the hero's journey that is Dennis Teston's class) for being my weekly sanity checkpoint through this writing process. To my therapist, Melissa Daum, for witnessing and guiding me through it all. To Lift Floats, for the creative downloads. To Dani Shapiro, for your writing advice, and for *Still Writing*. Nicole Jardim and Jenn Racioppi—my book-writing group, I can't imagine navigating this wild ride without you two. Thank you for listening to my late night voice texts during deadlines, and for your advice and loving support at every step. Joel Runyon—thank you for encouraging me, and reminding me that I can, in fact, do impossible things.

Gabby Bernstein, thank you for lighting the path for me for the past thirteen years. I wouldn't be who I am today without you. Dr. Frank Lipman, for your generosity and wisdom. Jamie Graber, for being my sounding board through it all. Jeanne Grabowski, for being the Glennon to my Liz (and the Liz to my Glennon). Jim Curtis, for your continuous support. Kirk Hensler, for putting up with my photo shoot antics (again). Bria Anderson, for the gift of Maria. To the Girlfriends text, and all of my friends and family—thank you for your love and support throughout this project.

To Dad, Mom, and Lisa: I love you more than words could ever say. Dad—your courage, strength, openness, and optimism have made this journey the most meaningful experience of my life. Mom—you are the ultimate caregiver. Thank you for your positivity, unwavering support, and dedication to our family. Lisa—thank you for always being by my side in this lifetime. You are my forever best friend.

To the Healthy Crush readers who have been with me since 2008, to the readers who share their experiences with me daily, and to you reading this now: thank you for being in my life.

BIBLIOGRAPHY

THE RENAISSANCE OF CANNABIS AND MUSHROOMS

Baum, Dan. "Legalize It All." *Harper's Magazine*, March 31, 2016. https://harpers.org/archive/2016/04/legalize-it-all/.

Brand, E. J., & Zhao, Z. (2017). "Cannabis in Chinese Medicine: Are Some Traditional Indications Referenced in Ancient Literature Related to Cannabinoids?" *Frontiers in Pharmacology* 8, 108. https://doi.org/10.3389/fphar.2017.00108.

Bridgeman, M. B., & Abazia, D. T. (2017). "Medicinal Cannabis: History, Pharmacology, and Implications for the Acute Care Setting." *P&T: A Peer-Reviewed Journal for Formulary Management* 42(3), 180–188.

Daniel, J., & Haberman, M. (2018). "Clinical Potential of Psilocybin as a Treatment for Mental Health Conditions." *The Mental Health Clinician* 7(1), 24–28. https://doi.org/10.9740/mhc.2017.01.024.

Iffland, K., & Grotenhermen, F. (2017). "An Update on Safety and Side Effects of Cannabidiol: A Review of Clinical Data and Relevant Animal Studies." *Cannabis and Cannabinoid Research* 2(1), 139–154. https://doi.org/10.1089/can.2016.0034.

King, R. S., & Mauer, M. (2006). "The War on Marijuana: The Transformation of the War on Drugs in the 1990s." *Harm Reduction Journal* 3, 6. https://doi.org/10.1186/1477-7517-3-6.

Lee, K. H., Morris-Natschke, S. L., Yang, X., Huang, R., Zhou, T., Wu, S. F., Shi, Q., & Itokawa, H. (2012). "Recent Progress of Research on Medicinal Mushrooms, Foods, and other Herbal Products Used in Traditional Chinese Medicine." *Journal of Traditional and Complementary Medicine* 2(2), 84–95.

Lindequist, U., Kim, H. W., Tiralongo, E., & Van Griensven, L. (2014). "Medicinal Mushrooms." *Evidence-Based Complementary and Alternative Medicine: eCAM*, 2014, 806180. https://doi.org/10.1155/2014/806180.

McKenna, G. J. (2014). "The Current Status of Medical Marijuana in the United States." *Hawai'i Journal of Medicine & Public Health: A Journal of Asia Pacific Medicine & Public Health* 73(4), 105–108.

Mead, A. (2019). "Legal and Regulatory Issues Governing Cannabis and Cannabis-Derived Products in the United States." *Frontiers in Plant Science* 10, 697. https://doi.org/10.3389/fpls.2019.00697.

Moore, L. D., & Elkavich, A. (2008). "Who's Using and Who's Doing Time: Incarceration, the War on Drugs, and Public Health. *American Journal of Public Health* 98(9 Suppl), S176—S180. https://doi.org/10.2105/ajph.98.supplement_1.s176.

National Academies of Sciences, Engineering, and Medicine. (2017). *The Health Effects of Cannabis and Cannabinoids: The Current State of Evidence and Recommendations for Research.* Washington (DC): National Academies Press (US), 15.

O'Shaughnessy, W. B. (1843). "On the Preparations of the Indian Hemp, or Gunjah: Cannabis Indica Their Effects on the Animal System in Health, and their Utility in the Treatment of Tetanus and other Convulsive Diseases." *Provincial Medical Journal and Retrospect of the Medical Sciences* 5(123), 363–369.

Stamets, P., & Zwickey, H. (2014). "Medicinal Mushrooms: Ancient Remedies Meet Modern Science." *Integrative Medicine* (Encinitas, CA) 13(1), 46–47.

Urits, I., Borchart, M., Hasegawa, M., Kochanski, J., Orhurhu, V., & Viswanath, O. (2019). "An Update of Current Cannabis-Based Pharmaceuticals in Pain Medicine." *Pain and Therapy* 8(1), 41–51. https://doi.org/10.1007/s40122-019-0114-4.

LET'S TALK ABOUT CANNABIS

Andre, C. M., Hausman, J. F., & Guerriero, G. (2016). "Cannabis Sativa: The Plant of the Thousand and One Molecules." *Frontiers in Plant Science* 7, 19. https://doi.org/10.3389/fpls.2016.00019.

Barcott, Bruce, Chant, Ian, & Downs, David. "Are You Getting the CBD You Paid for? We Put 47 Products to the Test." Leafly, January 22, 2020. https://www.leafly.com/news/strains-products/cbd-oil-test-results.

Bonn-Miller, M. O., Loflin, M., Thomas, B. F., Marcu, J. P., Hyke, T., & Vandrey, R. (2017). "Labeling Accuracy of Cannabidiol Extracts Sold Online." *JAMA* 318(17), 1708–1709. https://doi.org/10.1001/jama.2017.11909.

Bruni, N., Della Pepa, C., Oliaro-Bosso, S., Pessione, E., Gastaldi, D., & Dosio, F. (2018). "Cannabinoid Delivery Systems for Pain and Inflammation Treatment." *Molecules* (Basel, Switzerland) 23(10), 2478. https://doi.org/10.3390/molecules23102478.

Centers for Disease Control and Prevention (February 14, 2020). "Outbreak of Lung Injury Associated with the Use of E-Cigarette, or Vaping, Products. Centers for Disease Control and Prevention." https://www.cdc.gov/tobacco/basic_information/e-cigarettes/severe-lung-disease.html.

Colbin, Annemarie. *Food and Healing.* New York: Ballantine Books, 1996.

Corroon, J., & Kight, R. (2018). "Regulatory Status of Cannabidiol in the United States: A Perspective." *Cannabis and Cannabinoid Research* 3(1), 190–194. https://doi.org/10.1089/can.2018.0030.

D'Souza, D. C., Sewell, R. A., & Ranganathan, M. (2009). "Cannabis and Psychosis/Schizophrenia: Human Studies. *European Archives of Psychiatry and Clinical Neuroscience* 259(7), 413–431. https://doi.org/10.1007/s00406-009-0024-2.

Fuss, J., Bindila, L., Wiedemann, K., Auer, M. K., Briken, P., & Biedermann, S. V. (2017). "Masturbation to Orgasm Stimulates the Release of the Endocannabinoid 2-Arachidonoylglycerol in Humans." *The Journal of Sexual Medicine* 14(11), 1372–1379. doi: 10.1016/j.jsxm.2017.09.016.

Gamble, L. J., Boesch, J. M., Frye, C. W., Schwark, W. S., Mann, S., Wolfe, L., Brown, H., Berthelsen, E. S., & Wakshlag, J. J. (2018). "Pharmacokinetics, Safety, and Clinical Efficacy of Cannabidiol Treatment in Osteoarthritic Dogs." *Frontiers in Veterinary Science* 5, 165. https://doi.org/10.3389/fvets.2018.00165.

Gaoni, Y., & Mechoulam, R. (1964). "Isolation, Structure, and Partial Synthesis of an Active Constituent of Hashish." *Journal of the American Chemical Society* 86(8), 1646–1647. doi: 10.1021/ja01062a046.

Grant, K. S., Petroff, R., Isoherranen, N., Stella, N., & Burbacher, T. M. (2018). "Cannabis Use During Pregnancy: Pharmacokinetics and Effects on Child Development." *Pharmacology & Therapeutics* 182, 133–151. https://doi.org/10.1016/j.pharmthera.2017.08.014.

Huestis, M. A. (2007). "Human Cannabinoid Pharmacokinetics." *Chemistry & Biodiversity* 4(8), 1770–1804. https://doi.org/10.1002/cbdv.200790152.

Lemberger, L., Martz, R., Rodda, B., Forney, R., & Rowe, H. (1973). "Comparative Pharmacology of Δ9-Tetrahydrocannabinol and its Metabolite, 11-OH-Δ9-Tetrahydrocannabinol." *Journal of Clinical Investigation* 52(10), 2411–2417. doi: 10.1172/jci107431.

Lu, H. C., & Mackie, K. (2016). "An Introduction to the Endogenous Cannabinoid System." *Biological Psychiatry* 79(7), 516–525. https://doi.org/10.1016/j.biopsych.2015.07.028.

Maccallum, C. A., & Russo, E. B. (2018). "Practical Considerations in Medical Cannabis Administration and Dosing." *European Journal of Internal Medicine* 49, 12–19. doi: 10.1016/j.ejim.2018.01.004.

Mcgrath, S., Bartner, L. R., Rao, S., Packer, R. A., & Gustafson, D. L. (2019). "Randomized Blinded Controlled Clinical Trial to Assess the Effect of Oral Cannabidiol Administration in Addition to Conventional Antiepileptic Treatment on Seizure Frequency in Dogs with Intractable Idiopathic Epilepsy." *Journal of the American Veterinary Medical Association* 254(11), 1301–1308. doi: 10.2460/javma.254.11.1301.

Mcguire, P., Robson, P., Cubala, W. J., Vasile, D., Morrison, P. D., Barron, R., Taylor, A., & Wright, S. (2018). "Cannabidiol (CBD) as an Adjunctive Therapy in Schizophrenia: A Multicenter Randomized Controlled Trial." *American Journal of Psychiatry* 175(3), 225–231. doi: 10.1176/appi.ajp.2017.17030325.

Mechoulam, R., Fride, E., & Marzo, V. D. (1998). "Endocannabinoids." *European Journal of Pharmacology* 359(1), 1–18. doi: 10.1016/s0014-2999(98)00649-9.

Mechoulam, R., & Parker, L. A. (2013). "The Endocannabinoid System and the Brain." *Annual Review of Psychology* 64(1), 21–47. doi: 10.1146/annurev-psych-113011-143739.

Moreau, M., Ibeh, U., Decosmo, K., Bih, N., Yasmin-Karim, S., Toyang, N., Lowe, H., & Ngwa, W. (2019). "Flavonoid Derivative of Cannabis Demonstrates Therapeutic Potential in Preclinical Models of Metastatic Pancreatic Cancer." *Frontiers in Oncology* 9, 660. https://doi.org/10.3389/fonc.2019.00660.

Muller, C., Morales, P., & Reggio, P. H. (2019). "Cannabinoid Ligands Targeting TRP Channels." *Frontiers in Molecular Neuroscience* 11, 487. https://doi.org/10.3389/fnmol .2018.00487.

National Institute on Drug Abuse. (2019, January 29). "Overdose Death Rates." https:// www.drugabuse.gov/related-topics/trends-statistics/overdose-death-rates.

Project CBD. "Cannabis Oil Extraction Methods: How CBD Oil Is Made." https:// www.projectcbd.org/cbd-101/how-is-cbd-oil-made.

Russo, E. B. (2011). "Taming THC: Potential Cannabis Synergy and Phytocannabinoid-Terpenoid Entourage Effects." *British Journal of Pharmacology* 163(7), 1344–1364. https://doi.org/10.1111/j.1476-5381.2011.01238.x.

Russo, E. B. (2016). "Clinical Endocannabinoid Deficiency Reconsidered: Current Research Supports the Theory in Migraine, Fibromyalgia, Irritable Bowel, and Other Treatment-Resistant Syndromes." *Cannabis and Cannabinoid Research* 1(1), 154–165. doi: 10.1089/can.2016.0009.

Russo, E. B. (2019). "The Case for the Entourage Effect and Conventional Breeding of Clinical Cannabis: No 'Strain,' No Gain." *Frontiers in Plant Science* 9, 1969. https://doi .org/10.3389/fpls.2018.01969.

Russo, E. B., Burnett, A., Hall, B., & Parker, K. K. (2005). "Agonistic Properties of Cannabidiol at 5-HT1a Receptors." *Neurochemical Research* 30(8), 1037–1043. doi: 10.1007 /s11064-005-6978-1.

SC Labs. "Explore Cannabinoids." (2017, April 24). https://www.sclabs.com/cannabi noids/.

SC Labs. "Learn About Terpenes." (2017, April 24). https://www.sclabs.com/terpenes/.

Sharafi, G., He, H., & Nikfarjam, M. (2019). "Potential Use of Cannabinoids for the Treatment of Pancreatic Cancer." *Journal of Pancreatic Cancer* 5(1), 1–7. https://doi.org /10.1089/pancan.2018.0019.

Taha, T., Meiri, D., Talhamy, S., Wollner, M., Peer, A., & Bar-Sela, G. (2019). "Cannabis Impacts Tumor Response Rate to Nivolumab in Patients with Advanced Malignancies." *The Oncologist* 24(4), 549–554. doi: 10.1634/theoncologist.2018-0383.

Wang, M., Wang, Y. H., Avula, B., Radwan, M. M., Wanas, A. S., van Antwerp, J., Parcher, J. F., ElSohly, M. A., & Khan, I. A. (2016). "Decarboxylation Study of Acidic Cannabinoids: A Novel Approach Using Ultra-High-Performance Supercritical Fluid Chromatography/Photodiode Array-Mass Spectrometry." *Cannabis and Cannabinoid Research* 1(1), 262–271. https://doi.org/10.1089/can.2016.0020.

MEET THE MEDICINAL MUSHROOMS

Akramienė, D., Kondrotas, A., Didžiapetrienė, J., & Kėvelaitis, E. (November 2007). "Effects of ß-Glucans on the Immune System." *Medicina* 43(8), 597. https://doi.org/10 .3390/medicina43080076.

Baldauf, S. L., & Palmer, J. D. (1993). "Animals and Fungi Are Each Other's Closest Relatives: Congruent Rvidence from Multiple Proteins." *Proceedings of the National Academy of Sciences of the United States of America* 90(24), 11558–11562. https://doi.org /10.1073/pnas.90.24.11558.

Bashir, K., & Choi, J. S. (2017). "Clinical and Physiological Perspectives of β-Glucans: The Past, Present, and Future." *International Journal of Molecular Sciences* 18(9), 1906. https://doi.org/10.3390/ijms18091906.

Bastyr University (November 30, 2012). "FDA Approves Bastyr Turkey Tail Trial for Cancer Patients." https://bastyr.edu/news/general-news/2012/11/fda-approves-bastyr -turkey-tail-trial-cancer-patients.

Chan, G. C., Chan, W. K., & Sze, D. M. (2009). "The Effects of Beta-Glucan on Human Immune and Cancer Cells." *Journal of Hematology & Oncology* 2, 25. https://doi.org/10 .1186/1756-8722-2-25.

Chang, S.-T., & Wasser, S. P. (2012). "The Role of Culinary-Medicinal Mushrooms on Human Welfare with a Pyramid Model for Human Health." *International Journal of Medicinal Mushrooms* 14(2), 95–134. doi: 10.1615/intjmedmushr.v14.i2.10.

Four Sigmatic. "FAQ: Four Sigmatic Mushrooms." https://us.foursigmatic.com/faq.

Guggenheim, A. G., Wright, K. M., & Zwickey, H. L. (2014). "Immune Modulation from Five Major Mushrooms: Application to Integrative Oncology." *Integrative Medicine* (Encinitas, CA), 13(1), 32–44.

Host Defense. "FAQ: Host Defense Mushrooms." https://hostdefense.com/pages/faqs.

Kubo, K., Aoki, H., & Nanba, H. (1994). "Anti-diabetic Activity Present in the Fruit Body of Grifola frondosa (Maitake). I." *Biological & Pharmaceutical Bulletin* 17(8), 1106–1110. doi: 10.1248/bpb.17.1106.

Kulshreshtha, S., Mathur, N., & Bhatnagar, P. (2014). "Mushroom as a Product and Their Role in Mycoremediation." *AMB Express* 4, 29. https://doi.org/10.1186/s13568 -014-0029-8.

Lai, P-L, et al (2013). "Neurotrophic Properties of the Lion's Mane Medicinal Mushroom, *Hericium erinaceus* (Higher Basidiomycetes) from Malaysia." *International Journal of Medicinal Mushrooms* 15, 539-554. doi: 10.1615/IntJMedMushr.v15.i6.30.

Lindequist, U., Niedermeyer, T. H., & Jülich, W. D. (2005). "The Pharmacological Potential of Mushrooms." *Evidence-Based Complementary and Alternative Medicine: eCAM* 2(3), 285–299. https://doi.org/10.1093/ecam/neh107.

Phan, C.-W., David, P., Naidu, M., Wong, K.-H., & Sabaratnam, V. (2014). "Therapeutic Potential of Culinary-Medicinal Mushrooms for the Management of Neurodegenerative Diseases: Diversity, Metabolite, and Mechanism." *Critical Reviews in Biotechnology* 35(3), 355–368. doi: 10.3109/07388551.2014.887649.

Rogers, Robert. *The Fungal Pharmacy: the Complete Guide to Medicinal Mushrooms and Lichens of North America.* Berkeley, CA: North Atlantic Books, 2011.

Stamets, Paul. *Mycelium Running: How Mushrooms Can Help Save the World.* Berkeley, CA: Ten Speed Press, 2005.

Terakawa, N., Matsui, Y., Satoi, S., Yanagimoto, H., Takahashi, K., Yamamoto, T., Yamao, J., Takai, S., Kwon, A. H., & Kamiyama, Y. (2008). "Immunological Effect of Active Hexose Correlated Compound (AHCC) in Healthy Volunteers: A Double-Blind, Placebo-Controlled Trial." *Nutrition and Cancer* 60(5), 643–651. doi: 10.1080 /01635580801993280.

Tuli, H. S., Sandhu, S. S., & Sharma, A. K. (2014). "Pharmacological and Therapeutic Potential of Cordyceps with Special Reference to Cordycepin." *3 Biotech* 4(1), 1–12. https://doi.org/10.1007/s13205-013-0121-9.

Wachtel-Galor, S., Yuen, J., Buswell, J. A., et al. "*Ganoderma lucidum* (Lingzhi or Reishi): A Medicinal Mushroom," in Benzie, I. F. F., Wachtel-Galor, S., editors. *Herbal Medicine: Biomolecular and Clinical Aspects*, second edition. Boca Raton: CRC Press/Taylor & Francis; 2011. Available from: https://www.ncbi.nlm.nih.gov/books /NBK92757/.

Wasser, S.P. (2002). "Medicinal Mushrooms as a Source of Antitumor and Immunomodulating Polysaccharides." *Applied Microbiology and Biotechnology* 60(3), 258–274. doi: 10 .1007/s00253-002-1076-7.

Wasser, S. P. (2017). "Medicinal Mushrooms in Human Clinical Studies. Part I. Anticancer, Oncoimmunological, and Immunomodulatory Activities: A Review." *International Journal of Medicinal Mushrooms* 19(4), 279–317. doi: 10.1615/intjmedmushrooms.v19 .i4.10.

Weil, A. (2019, June 10). "Ask Dr. Weil: Is It Safe to Eat Raw Mushrooms?" https:// www.prevention.com/health/a20442817/ask-dr-weil-is-it-true-that-you-should-never -eat-mushrooms-raw/

Wolfe, D. (2012). *Chaga: King of the Medicinal Mushrooms*. Berkeley, CA: North Atlantic Books.

DEEPEN YOUR SLEEP

Babson, K. A., Sottile, J., & Morabito, D. (2017). "Cannabis, Cannabinoids, and Sleep: A Review of the Literature." *Current Psychiatry Reports* 19(4). doi: 10.1007/s11920-017 -0775-9.

Besedovsky, L., Lange, T., & Born, J. (2012). "Sleep and Immune Function." *Pflugers Archive: European Journal of Physiology* 463(1), 121–137. https://doi.org/10.1007/s00424 -011-1044-0.

Blessing, E. M., Steenkamp, M. M., Manzanares, J., & Marmar, C. R. (2015). "Cannabidiol as a Potential Treatment for Anxiety Disorders." *Neurotherapeutics: The Journal of the American Society for Experimental NeuroTherapeutics* 12(4), 825–836. https://doi.org /10.1007/s13311-015-0387-1.

Cui, X.Y., Cui, S.-Y., Zhang, J., Wang, Z.-J., Yu, B., Sheng, Z.-F., Zhang, X.-Q., Zhang, Y.-H. (2012). "Extract of *Ganoderma lucidum* Prolongs Sleep Time in Rats." *Journal of Ethnopharmacology* 139(3), 796–800. doi: 10.1016/j.jep.2011.12.020.

Liao, L. Y., He, Y. F., Li, L., Meng, H., Dong, Y. M., Yi, F., & Xiao, P. G. (2018). "A Preliminary Review of Studies on Adaptogens: Comparison of Their Bioactivity in TCM with that of Ginseng-like Herbs Used Worldwide. *Chinese Medicine* 13, 57. https://doi .org/10.1186/s13020-018-0214-9.

Papagianni, E. P., & Stevenson, C. W. (2019). "Cannabinoid Regulation of Fear and Anxiety: An Update." *Current Psychiatry Reports* 21(6), 38. https://doi.org/10.1007/s11920 -019-1026-z.

Project CBD: Medical Marijuana & Cannabinoid Science (October 29, 2017). "Cannabis & Sleep Disturbances." https://www.projectcbd.org/medicine/cannabis-sleep -disturbances.

EASE YOUR PAIN

Bouaziz, J., Bar On, A., Seidman, D. S., & Soriano, D. (2017). "The Clinical Significance of Endocannabinoids in Endometriosis Pain Management." *Cannabis and Cannabinoid Research* 2(1), 72–80. https://doi.org/10.1089/can.2016.0035.

Center for Drug Evaluation and Research. (n.d.). Ibuprofen Drug Facts Label. https:// www.fda.gov/drugs/postmarket-drug-safety-information-patients-and-providers /ibuprofen-drug-facts-label.

Kaufman, D. W., Kelly, J. P., Battista, D. R., Malone, M. K., Weinstein, R. B., & Shiffman, S. (2018). "Exceeding the Daily Dosing Limit of Nonsteroidal Anti-inflammatory Drugs Among Ibuprofen Uusers. *Pharmacoepidemiology and Drug Safety* 27(3), 322–331. doi: 10.1002/pds.4391.

Miller, Sara G. (June 6, 2017). "Marijuana for Menstrual Cramps? New York Considers Medical Option." Live Science. Retrieved from https://www.livescience.com/59370 -marijuana-period-cramps-dysmenorrhea.html.

Pazzi, F., Fabero, R. F. (2017) "Effects of *Ganoderma lucidum* on Pain in Women with Fibromyalgia." *Fibromyalgia Open Access* 2, 115.

Sanodiya, B., Thakur, G., Baghel, R., Prasad, G., & Bisen, P. (2009). "*Ganoderma lucidum*: A Potent Pharmacological Macrofungus." *Current Pharmaceutical Biotechnology* 10(8), 717–742. doi: 10.2174/138920109789978757.

Vučković, S., Srebro, D., Vujović, K. S., Vučetić, Č., & Prostran, M. (2018). "Cannabinoids and Pain: New Insights from Old Molecules." *Frontiers in Pharmacology* 9, 1259. https://doi.org/10.3389/fphar.2018.01259.

Wiese, B., & Wilson-Poe, A. R. (2018). "Emerging Evidence for Cannabis' Role in Opioid Use Disorder." *Cannabis and Cannabinoid Research* 3(1), 179–189. https://doi.org /10.1089/can.2018.0022.

CALM STRESS AND ANXIETY

Ryu, S., Kim, H. G., Kim, J. Y., Kim, S. Y., & Cho, K.-O. (2018). "*Hericium erinaceus* Extract Reduces Anxiety and Depressive Behaviors by Promoting Hippocampal Neurogenesis in the Adult Mouse Brain." *Journal of Medicinal Food* 21(2), 174–180. doi: 10 .1089/jmf.2017.4006.

Zhao, H., Zhang, Q., Zhao, L., Huang, X., Wang, J., & Kang, X. (2012). "Spore Powder of *Ganoderma lucidum* Improves Cancer-Related Fatigue in Breast Cancer Patients Undergoing Endocrine Therapy: A Pilot Clinical Trial." *Evidence-Based Complementary and Alternative Medicine* 2012, 1–8. doi: 10.1155/2012/809614.

INCREASE YOUR ENERGY, ENHANCE YOUR FOCUS, UPLIFT YOUR MOOD

Huang, W. J., Chen, W. W., & Zhang, X. (2016). "Endocannabinoid System: Role in Depression, Reward and Pain Control (Review)." *Molecular Medicine Reports* 14(4), 2899–2903. https://doi.org/10.3892/mmr.2016.5585.

Le Foll, B., Gorelick, D. A., & Goldberg, S. R. (2009). "The Future of Endocannabinoid-Oriented Clinical Research After CB1 Antagonists. *Psychopharmacology* 205(1), 171–174. https://doi.org/10.1007/s00213-009-1506-7.

Pandey, R., Mousawy, K., Nagarkatti, M., & Nagarkatti, P. (2009). "Endocannabinoids and Immune Regulation." *Pharmacological Research* 60(2), 85–92. https://doi.org/10.1016/j.phrs.2009.03.019

Prenderville, J. A., Kelly, Á. M., & Downer, E. J. (2015). "The Role of Cannabinoids in Adult Neurogenesis." *British Journal of Pharmacology* 172(16), 3950–3963. https://doi.org/10.1111/bph.13186.

SUPERCHARGE YOUR SEX DRIVE

Androvicova, R., Horacek, J., Stark, T., Drago, F., & Micale, V. (2017). "Endocannabinoid System in Sexual Motivational Processes: Is It a Novel Therapeutic Horizon?" *Pharmacological Research* 115, 200–208. doi: 10.1016/j.phrs.2016.11.021.

Lin, B., & Li, S. "Cordyceps as an Herbal Drug," in Benzie, I. F. F., Wachtel-Galor, S., editors, *Herbal Medicine: Biomolecular and Clinical Aspects*, second edition. Boca Raton: CRC Press/Taylor & Francis; 2011. Available from: https://www.ncbi.nlm.nih.gov/books/NBK92758/.

Lynn, B. K., López, J. D., Miller, C., Thompson, J., & Campian, E. C. (2019). "The Relationship between Marijuana Use Prior to Sex and Sexual Function in Women." *Sexual Medicine* 7(2), 192–197. https://doi.org/10.1016/j.esxm.2019.01.003.

Panda, A. K., & Swain, K. C. (2011). "Traditional Uses and Medicinal Potential of Cordyceps Sinensis of Sikkim." *Journal of Ayurveda and Integrative Medicine* 2(1), 9–13. https://doi.org/10.4103/0975-9476.78183.

NOURISH YOUR SKIN

Sheriff, T., Lin, M. J., Dubin, D., & Khorasani, H. (2019). "The Potential Role of Cannabinoids in Dermatology." *Journal of Dermatological Treatment*, 1–7. doi: 10.1080/09546634.2019.1675854.

Yun, J. S., Pahk, J. W., Lee, J. S., Shin, W. C., Lee, S. Y., & Hong, E. K. (2011). "*Inonotus obliquus* Protects Against Oxidative Stress-induced Apoptosis and Premature Senescence." *Molecules and Cells* 31(5), 423–429. https://doi.org/10.1007/s10059-011-0256-7.

Wang, J., Cao, B., Zhao, H., & Feng, J. (2017). "Emerging Roles of *Ganoderma Lucidum* in Anti-Aging." *Aging and Disease* 8(6), 691–707. https://doi.org/10.14336/AD.2017.0410.

CANNABIS AND CANCER

Abrams, D. I. (2016). "Integrating Cannabis into Clinical Cancer Care." *Current Oncology* (Toronto) 23(2), S8—S14. https://doi.org/10.3747/co.23.3099

Bienenstock, D. (February 6, 2019). "A Patient's Guide to Using Cannabis for Cancer." https://www.leafly.com/news/health/how-to-use-medical-marijuana-for-cancer.

Dariš, B., Tancer Verboten, M., Knez, Ž., & Ferk, P. (2019). "Cannabinoids in Cancer Treatment: Therapeutic Potential and Legislation." *Bosnian Journal of Basic Medical Sciences* 19(1), 14–23. https://doi.org/10.17305/bjbms.2018.3532.

National Cancer Institute. "Cannabis and Cannabinoids." https://www.cancer.gov /about-cancer/treatment/cam/hp/cannabis-pdq.

National Institute on Drug Abuse. "Marijuana as Medicine." https://www.drugabuse .gov/publications/drugfacts/marijuana-medicine.

The Realm of Caring. "Cancer Cannabis Dosing Guidelines." http://www.theroc.us /images/CancerDosing.pdf.

Sharafi, G., He, H., & Nikfarjam, M. (2019). "Potential Use of Cannabinoids for the Treatment of Pancreatic Cancer." *Journal of Pancreatic Cancer* 5(1), 1–7. https://doi.org /10.1089/pancan.2018.0019.

Yasmin-Karim, S., Moreau, M., Mueller, R., Sinha, N., Dabney, R., Herman, A., & Ngwa, W. (2018). "Enhancing the Therapeutic Efficacy of Cancer Treatment With Cannabinoids." *Frontiers in Oncology* 8, 114. https://doi.org/10.3389/fonc.2018.00114.

MEDICINAL MUSHROOMS AND CANCER

Aleem, E. (2013). "β -Glucans and their Applications in Cancer Therapy: Focus on Human Studies." *Anti-Cancer Agents in Medicinal Chemistry* 13(5), 709–719. doi: 10 .2174/1871520611313050005

Blagodatski, A., Yatsunskaya, M., Mikhailova, V., Tiasto, V., Kagansky, A., & Katanaev, V. L. (2018). "Medicinal Mushrooms as an Attractive New Source of Natural Compounds for Future Cancer Therapy." *Oncotarget* 9(49), 29259–29274. https://doi.org/10 .18632/oncotarget.25660.

Konno, S. (2009). "Synergistic Potentiation of D-fraction with Vitamin C as Possible Alternative Approach for Cancer Therapy." *International Journal of General Medicine* 2, 91–108. https://doi.org/10.2147/ijgm.s5498.

Król, S. K., Kiełbus, M., Rivero-Müller, A., & Stepulak, A. (2015). "Comprehensive Review on Betulin as a Potent Anticancer Agent." *BioMed Research International* 2015, 584189. https://doi.org/10.1155/2015/584189.

Lee, H. S., Kim, E. J., & Kim, S. H. (2015). "Ethanol Extract of Innotus Obliquus (Chaga mushroom) Induces G1 Cell Cycle Arrest in HT-29 Human Colon Cancer Cells." *Nutrition Research and Practice* 9(2), 111–116. https://doi.org/10.4162/nrp.2015.9.2.111.

PDQ Integrative, Alternative, and Complementary Therapies Editorial Board (January 17, 2019). "Medicinal Mushrooms (PDQ®): Patient Version," in *PDQ Cancer Information Summaries*. Bethesda (MD): National Cancer Institute. https://www.ncbi.nlm .nih.gov/books/NBK424937/.

Torkelson, C. J., Sweet, E., Martzen, M. R., Sasagawa, M., Wenner, C. A., Gay, J., Putiri, A., & Standish, L. J. (2012). "Phase 1 Clinical Trial of Trametes Versicolor in Women with Breast Cancer." *ISRN Oncology* 2012, 251632. https://doi.org/10.5402/2012/251632.

Wasser, S. (2014). "Medicinal Mushroom Science: Current Perspectives, Advances, Evidences, and Challenges." *Biomedical Journal* 37(6), 345. doi: 10.4103/2319-4170.138318.

Zhang, M., Zhang, Y., Zhang, L., & Tian, Q. (2019). "Mushroom Polysaccharide Lentinan for Treating Different Types of Cancers: A Review of 12 Years Clinical Studies in China." *Progress in Molecular Biology and Translational Science Glycans and Glycosaminoglycans as Clinical Biomarkers and Therapeutics—Part B*, 297–328. doi: 10.1016/bs.pmbts.2019.02.013.

OTHER ADVANCED CASES

Elms, L., Shannon, S., Hughes, S., & Lewis, N. (2019). "Cannabidiol in the Treatment of Post-Traumatic Stress Disorder: A Case Series." *Journal of Alternative and Complementary Medicine* 25(4), 392–397. https://doi.org/10.1089/acm.2018.0437.

Mithoefer, M. C., Feduccia, A. A., Jerome, L., Mithoefer, A., Wagner, M., Walsh, Z., Hamilton, S., Yazar-Klosinski, B., Emerson, A., & Doblin, R. (2019). "MDMA-Assisted Psychotherapy for Treatment of PTSD: Study Design and Rationale for Phase 3 Trials Based on Pooled Analysis of Six Phase 2 Randomized Controlled Trials." *Psychopharmacology* 236(9), 2735–2745. https://doi.org/10.1007/s00213-019-05249-5.

Neumeister, A., Normandin, M. D., Pietrzak, R. H., Piomelli, D., Zheng, M. Q., Gujarro-Anton, A., Potenza, M. N., Bailey, C. R., Lin, S. F., Najafzadeh, S., Ropchan, J., Henry, S., Corsi-Travali, S., Carson, R. E., & Huang, Y. (2013). "Elevated Brain Cannabinoid CB1 Receptor Availability in Post-traumatic Stress Disorder: A Positron Emission Tomography Study." *Molecular Psychiatry* 18(9), 1034–1040. https://doi.org/10.1038/mp.2013.61.

Perucca, E. (2017). "Cannabinoids in the Treatment of Epilepsy: Hard Evidence at Last?" *Journal of Epilepsy Research* 7(2), 61–76. https://doi.org/10.14581/jer.17012.

MAGIC MUSHROOMS: THE CASE FOR PSILOCYBIN

Carhart-Harris, R. L., Bolstridge, M., Day, C., Rucker, J., Watts, R., Erritzoe, D. E., Kaelen, M., Giribaldi, B., Bloomfield, M., Pilling, S., Rickard, J. A., Forbes, B., Feilding, A., Taylor, D., Curran, H. V., & Nutt, D. J. (2018). "Psilocybin with Psychological Support for Treatment-Resistant Depression: Six-Month Follow-Up." *Psychopharmacology* 235(2), 399–408. https://doi.org/10.1007/s00213-017-4771-x.

Carhart-Harris, R. L., & Goodwin, G. M. (2017). "The Therapeutic Potential of Psychedelic Drugs: Past, Present, and Future." *Neuropsychopharmacology: Official Publication of the American College of Neuropsychopharmacology* 42(11), 2105–2113. https://doi.org/10.1038/npp.2017.84.

Griffiths, R. R., Johnson, M. W., Carducci, M. A., Umbricht, A., Richards, W. A., Richards, B. D., Cosimano, M. P., & Klinedinst, M. A. (2016). "Psilocybin Produces Substantial and Sustained Decreases in Depression and Anxiety in Patients with Life-threatening Cancer: A Randomized Double-blind Trial." *Journal of Psychopharmacology* 30(12), 1181–1197. https://doi.org/10.1177/0269881116675513.

Haze, V., & Mandrake, K. (2016). *The Psilocybin Mushroom Bible.* Toronto, Canada: Green Candy Press.

Prochazkova, L., Lippelt, D. P., Colzato, L. S., Kuchar, M., Sjoerds, Z., & Hommel, B. (2018). "Exploring the Effect of Microdosing Psychedelics on Creativity in an Open-Label Natural Setting." *Psychopharmacology* 235(12), 3401–3413. https://doi.org/10.1007/s00213-018-5049-7.

"The Safety and Efficacy of Psilocybin in Participants With Treatment Resistant Depression—Full Text View." (n.d.). Retrieved from https://clinicaltrials.gov/ct2/show/NCT03775200.

The Third Wave. "The Ultimate Guide to Psilocybin Mushrooms." https://thethird-wave.co/psychedelics/shrooms/

GENERAL INDEX

Note: Page numbers in *italics* indicate recipes. *See also* **Index of Recipes**

anxiety and, 197–198

beta-glucans in, 87, 90–91, 105, 120, 223, 273

buying, 95–96

cancer and, 273–276

carcinogens in, 99

chemo side effects and, 280, 286–287, *292*, *293*, *294–297*

choosing products, 96–98

consuming options, 93–94

cooked vs. raw, 98–99

cooking with, 153, 210–211, 224

cost considerations, 100–101

daily rituals using, 243–245

defined, 89

delivery methods, 175, 198, 210–211

doctor consult about alternative therapies and, 257–262

dosing, 101–103

drug interactions precaution, 276

for energy, focus, and mood, 210–211, *212–213*, *215–218*, *219–220*

extracting medicine from, 91–92

foraging in the wild for, 101

fruiting body vs. mycelium, 96–98

as fungi, not plants, 86

healing benefits, 105–106, 111

health of the planet and, 86

immunity and, 223–224, *228–229*

magic mushrooms vs., 92 (*See also* mushrooms, psychedelic (psilocybin))

medicinal properties, 89–90

medicine inside, 90–92

mycelium-based products, 96–97, 98

organic importance, 99–100

other conditions and, 303–306

others to watch, 128

pain and, 189–191

psychoactive effects and, 129

resources, 323–324, 325

rise of, 7–8

scientific names of, 92–93

sex drive and, 232–233, *234*

skincare and, 241–*242*

sources for, 95–96, 322–323

as "superfoods," 8

mushrooms, psychedelic (psilocybin), 307–319

current research, 308, 309–311

defined, 308

doses in research, 311–312

how psilocybin works, 311

importance of set, setting and intention, 318–319

libido and, 233

medicinal mushrooms vs., 92

microdosing, 312–318

potential uses for, 308

renaissance of, 7

resources, 325

treatment-resistant depression and, 306

mycelium, 86–87, 88

myrcene, 31–32, 174, 178

nano-emulsion/water-soluble CBD, 52–53

nerve pain/neuropathy, 183, 189–190, 210, 298, 299

nootropics, 212

oat straw, 198

oncologist, consulting about alternative therapies, 257–262

INDEX OF RECIPES

Note: Page numbers in *italics* indicate recipes.

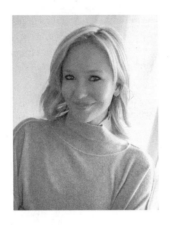

ABOUT THE AUTHOR

Jenny Sansouci is a writer; health coach, and the creator of the wellness blog Healthy Crush, where she's been writing for over a decade. She is a graduate of the Institute for Integrative Nutrition, and has been trained by functional medicine doctor Frank Lipman, MD in New York City. She is based in Brooklyn, New York.

STAY CONNECTED:

Instagram: @jennysansouci
Twitter: @jennysansouci
Blog: HealthyCrush.com
Facebook: Healthy Crush
Book Resources and Updates: RebelsApothecary.com